VOICELESS CHILD

No one dreamed she might survive, might talk.
Except two ordinary people ...

Ann Widick Giganti

Table of Contents

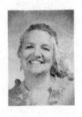

Ann Giganti

Cover designed by Ann Giganti

Author note: All is true. Some names have been changed.

Ann Widick Giganti
Visit my website at www.voicelesschild.com

Printed in the United States of America

First Printing: October 2017
Ann Widick Giganti

ISBN-978-0-9996064-2-1

*To all the amazing people who have graced my life
and assisted in the miracle of Heather
and the writing of this book*

*Family, especially James Gregory Giganti
Friends, especially Celeste and Mark Hoffenberg*

*Pediatric surgeons, especially Dr. Bruce Robert Maddern,
and the American Society of Pediatric Otolaryngology
(ASPO)*

*Mentors, especially Dr. Floyd Livingston,
Dr. David Geller,
Dr. Al Torres, Dr. Mahesh Soni*

*Editors, especially Julia Lee Dulfer,
Hilary Ross, Bev Katz Rosenbaum,
and Donna Chesher*

*Those who foster universal brotherhood
especially the Nirankari Mission*

*Those who promote music, theater, and the arts
especially Rosie's Theater Kids.*

Foreword

We all have heroes in our lives—Ann and Heather are two of mine.

My part in this story is that of the surgeon, one of a team that cared for Heather. Surgeons often try to shield themselves, but it is impossible to remain unemotional about this story of unconditional love. I met Heather when she was a toddler, and remember her quiet strength and infectious smile. She'd survived the worst that life can throw at a newborn baby.

Medical professionals often fail to recognize the struggles a family undergoes with an ill or special-needs child, let alone comprehend why a couple would volunteer to adopt one. Ann and Jim's determination to help an abandoned child is relevant to anyone's life. It is an example of working through dark times and not focusing on the difficult moments.

Endless patience, numerous doctor visits, therapies, and hard work are required for each small success and tenuous progress toward an uncertain future. Hope abounds that the child may become healthy and independent, but reality is too often peppered with disappointment, crushed dreams, and strained relationships.

The specialty of pediatric otolaryngology (children's ear, nose, and throat disorders) is a relatively new one. Greater numbers of premature babies were surviving in our nation's first neonatal intensive care units. Airway damage was one of their sentinel problems. From a small meeting of visionaries, we have grown to over three hundred dedicated surgeons. With the fortitude of giants, pioneers, such as Drs. Charles Bluestone, Sylvan Stool, and Robin Cotton, pushed through the envelope of what had once been considered surgically unachievable.

Families like the Gigantis pleaded for new cures, rightly so, to achieve greater normalcy. They refuted the notion that a child would never have a voice and refused the idea of condemning any youngster to a long-term future of breathing tubes and ventilators.

Voiceless Child kindles the fragile pilot lights of other families searching for their own success stories. It energizes the tireless professionals striving to discover solutions to the still unresolved puzzles of the many debilitating illnesses.

Doctors and medical teams sometimes take too much credit for a child's progress. The children and their families are the ones who deserve ongoing courtesy and abundant accolades.

Enjoy the story of Heather and how her dreams come true.

Dr. Bruce Robert Maddern
Pediatric Otolaryngologist   Jacksonville, Florida
President 2017-2018, American Society of Pediatric Otolaryngology (ASPO)

CHAPTER 1]
DORMANT SPIRIT

The baby's chest heaved as she struggled to breathe. Heather wasn't my child, but her distress tattered my heart. Fourteen months old, the little bundle lay swaddled in a blanket, forgotten and lost among unchanging medical routines.

"Just be glad she's only abandoned, not abused." The words on the other end of the phone line stung. I wrestled with anger, but instinct quieted any sharp response. The ribs of the dining-room chair pressed ridges into my back. My mind and muscles tensed, threatening to undo my feigned serenity. Anxiously I wove the phone cord in and out between my fingers and looped it around my thumb.

The laughter of my young son interrupted thoughts of the fragile girl and her dismal existence. Robust three-year-old Tony pushed his wooden tugboat around on the kitchen's vinyl floor, cresting the waves of his make-believe ocean.

Straightening my posture, I stirred my cup of strong coffee and took a quick sip and resumed the phone conversation.

"Don't you know about her?" I asked the social worker on the phone line. Sweet words flowed from my mouth. "The nurse said you'd guide my husband and me on how to proceed."

4

"I can't help," the woman repeated in blunt terms. She meant she wouldn't. I'd seen her, clipboard in hand, jotting crisp notes on a pad while talking to parents of ill children.

"Health and Rehabilitative Services says they'll speed up our licensing as foster or adoptive parents if you give the directive," I persisted.

"We don't need you," she replied. "There are others already licensed."

I halted the entreaty, baffled at her disinterest.

Didn't the woman realize what *abandoned* meant? Heather had never felt the warmth of the sun, seen a field of wild flowers, or smelled bacon and eggs sizzling in a skillet. She knew the pain of needles and surgery, but not the comfort of a mother's love, bedtime stories, and good-night kisses. Nor did she know the pleasure of a father's romping playfulness and gentle teasing.

Most hospital staff deemed Heather deaf, blind, and retarded. She did not know how to move her feet or hold up her head. Born ten weeks early, tiny enough to fit in the palms of two hands—breathing difficulties and resultant airway damage had silenced all her crying. Though the mute child teetered near death, a surgeon repetitively attempted fixing her airway. Certainly no one believed she would ever talk. No one dared dream she might survive to adulthood and have children of her own.

More visions of Heather flashed through my mind. She had lived her whole life in that hospital. The little one languished in a crib. She weighed just twelve pounds. Her skin had a bluish translucence; her face was puffy. Her body was limp as in sleep, but her eyes were open, not alert, yet not vacant. A sprinkling of fine brown hair lay flat on her head. A sterile, windowless room was her entire world. No one had ever taken her home. Rumor was they were transferring her to an institution.

If I'd had any idea of how that pitiful youngster was to transform our future, I would have shouted from the rooftop in fear and joy and disbelief. Somehow she'd summoned me and communicated an awareness of her plight.

At age eighteen, I had made a vow: no one in my family would ever be warehoused. *Institution.* The word brought sharp, twisting anguish. As a college freshman I volunteered in a state hospital . . . long, anonymous rows of children, handled only for assembly-line diaper and linen changes. Oh, the utter desolation and misery of those aloof, deformed babies, the helmet-wearing, head-banging children.

No one deserves such a fate, yet among them had been two who didn't seem to belong, as they could respond and communicate. Jenny's cerebral palsy imprisoned her clear mind in a malfunctioning body. Eddie was retarded and afflicted with waist-down paralysis. Both were in wheelchairs; both were gentle and loving. What they needed was a home and family. I don't know what happened to them.

Most disturbing was an eerie absence of the human spirit. Any child not already brain dead would suffer a living death in such a place. On the long city bus ride home, I'd mentally castigate those who'd orchestrated the children's dismal existence, while only superficially acknowledging the potentially greater tragic impact of caring for such a burden-laden child in one's home.

My life was simple until that warm September day. It started pleasantly enough with all the signs of an ordinary one in sunny Florida. The alarm clock buzzed, and my eight-year-old daughter, Jamie, tumbled out of bed. Her shoulder-length ringlets puffed out in disarray. A knock on the door signaled the school car pool's arrival.

We lived in Gainesville off a main road on the west side of town where the city ended and hardwood forest began. Early evening, the gravelly noise of tires rolling onto our driveway made me look out the window as my neighbor, Celeste, blared the horn of her sporty Toyota Celica. I went out to greet her. She lived two houses down and across the street with her husband, Mark, and daughter, Haley.

"Come with me to the hospital?" Celeste asked, making clear the reason for her sudden arrival. "Maria needs company, and I'm scared to see the sick babies." Maria lived nearby. Her newborn son had just been admitted to the PICU in heart failure. Maria, Celeste, and I were good friends.

The elderly woman at the hospital's front lobby desk handed over the visitor badges. Elevator doors opened, and we walked down the hallway to the pediatric intensive-care unit (PICU). Up one more floor would have led us to where I worked as a registered nurse in labor and delivery.

I inched open the door and called out to one of the PICU staff. After granting permission, an aide led us to a sink where we scrubbed our hands with germicidal soap.

Eerie whooshing from the ventilators and beeping of alarms broke the otherwise stifling silence. Six cribs were spaced along the perimeter of the circular room. We passed a baby dressed in pink, with so many wires and tubes attached to her that she looked like a marionette.

Adjacent to the next crib, our friend Maria sat in a sturdy wooden rocker with her ailing newborn son nestled to her chest. She rhythmically pulsed her feet to the floor to create a gentle sway.

Celeste glanced over at the baby in pink. "What's wrong with her?" she asked.

"No one's mentioned anything," Maria answered.

7

"She looks like a pulmonary kid," I said, after the briefest appraisal, not wanting to know more. Familiarity with the appearance of chronic lung patients had become second nature. As a new graduate, I'd worked the graveyard shift on a respiratory floor. The assignment was not voluntary; coughing and mucous made me queasy.

"Her name is Heather. She was born premature, and her lungs are damaged," confirmed the nurse.

"How old is she?" Celeste asked.

"Fourteen months."

"She's so tiny." Celeste winced.

"All her energy goes toward survival, not enough left for growing," the nurse said.

"Where's her family?" Celeste asked.

"She doesn't have one. Her mother never visits and doesn't want her."

Tears welled up in Celeste's eyes, "How could anyone discard a sick child?"

Amazed at my friend's naiveté, I handed her a tissue and conceded that my work in labor and delivery shielded me from such misfortunes. I related how I'd asked a neonatal nurse about how she coped with castaway babies. "Hmm, I don't have to face that sorrow. Sick newborns aren't much different from healthy ones," she'd explained. "It's after they go home or to PICU and the permanence of handicaps becomes more obvious, that is when they are abandoned."

Back in the PICU a few days later, I kept Maria company. Her baby would likely remain hospitalized for weeks. He needed surgery.

I observed as a plump nurse lifted the pulmonary kid out of the crib. Poor thing sagged limp like a rag doll. The nurse gently slid the small one into a swing and secured a safety belt. Even so, little

Heather slumped to one side. The caring woman tucked a fluffy teddy bear around the baby's belly and torso to serve as a propping bolster. She adjusted the flow of the supplemental oxygen and fiddled with life-monitors and double-checked that the warning alarms remained toggled on.

After she left, a young volunteer squatted beside the mirage of a child, attempting in vain to get a response. First he jiggled a brightly colored rattle. He cajoled and cheered, yet little Heather's face remained expressionless. He wound up a music box and attached it to the swing. She paid no attention.

"You don't like the music?" he asked. "Maybe this will spring a smile." His jovial face became a living cartoon. His cheeks puffed in and out like those of a blowfish. Eyebrows rippled; ears sprouted thumbs and waggling fingers. Heather's eyes stayed dull and her face remained barren.

"Some of the staff presume she has no vision, hearing, or thinking," he remarked, "but I keep trying." He walked from the room in quiet reflection.

A few minutes later erratic movements of the sorrowful pulmonary baby caught my eye. No longer resting passively in the baby swing, she pitched her head from side to side, in a weird total absence of uttering any sound. Her body jerked, arms and legs flailing. Seizure! I presumed. After starting for the emergency cord, I noticed the tracheotomy tube protruding from a hole in her neck.

"Maria, she isn't convulsing; she is crying!" The mental gear of a calm response to an emergency shifted to empathy. I moved closer to the little one with sudden comprehension of her strange quiet. Breathing in and out of the trach tube diverted all air from flowing through her vocal cords, making audible cries or giggles impossible.

"It is okay." I whispered soothing words to the anguished baby and touched her pale fingers. The weeping stopped. As I studied her face, our eyes met for an almost imperceptible fleeting moment, and her soul gripped mine. What gifts might lie hidden in her dormant spirit? Were the damning medical prophecies true?

"Why did she get the trach?" I asked the nurse.

"Premature babies tire and often stop breathing," she answered and explained further. To keep tiny babies alive until they grow bigger and stronger, a slender plastic airway is inserted via the mouth into the trachea. An electrical ventilator puffs breaths into their fragile lungs. In Heather's case, movement of the far end of that tube rubbed and abraded the delicate tissues of her trachea. The inevitable scarring obstructed most of her airway. To bypass the suffocating blockage, a pediatric surgeon cut an opening below the scarring and inserted the plastic tracheotomy tube.

I massaged Heather's forehead and slowly glided my fingers through her wispy hair until she drifted off to sleep. A spiritual sense goaded me and an idea crystallized: she was smart and deserved parents and a home. My preferred inclination is passivity, but in those initial moments of meeting her, I was ready to fight.

My composure slipped as I visualized images of the horrors of Heather's life and future. Overworked staff rely on a patient's family to perform minor nursing duties and bestow tender loving care because critical medical tasks take priority. What if there wasn't a family? Who would notice silent weeping? No mournful wail compels kind attentiveness. Heather's trach often plugged on her own secretions until suffocation caused her heart to slow enough to trigger an alarm.

Pediatric intensive care units aren't meant to have lifelong boarders. The PICU nurses told me Heather's biological mother had visited once or twice; that was all. They didn't say anything about her.

A poster urged interested couples to become foster parents for medically complex babies. I never knew of such things. For a year, they'd tried to find foster parents for Heather. No takers.

On the way home, I stopped to swim laps at a community pool, hoping to burn off a building anxiety and regain a cheery disposition.

Wet hair wrapped in a towel, I paced the sidewalk to the front door of our home. Without any contemplation of possible repercussions to my family, and quite unlike my usual studious scrutiny, I woke Jim who was asleep on the sofa. Although he hadn't been feeling well, I blurted out: "There's this baby, perhaps we could be her temporary mom and dad." I shared the little information that I knew. "Heather can't talk, and it is likely a permanent affliction."

My shocked husband rolled over and juxtaposed his back to block me. He tried becoming invisible by pulling a blanket up and covering his head.enhanced my efforts.

"Absolutely no," Jim mumbled in response to my preposterous proposal.

"But you said we could have as many children as I wanted," I said.

"Then I said two were enough. Never did we discuss taking in other people's children."

I brought him a glass of milk and a second blanket, then I went to bed.

CHAPTER 2] VOLATILE EMOTIONS

Thoughts of Heather's placement in a state institution piled up, entangling me in an emotional briar patch. Becoming her temporary parents seemed crazy to my husband, as he'd conjured an actual awareness of the many real-life consequences of such a rash decision. Jim and I thought we were done having children. Our son, Tony, had threatened a too-early birth. The doctor had confined me to bed for months.

Despite my enthusiasm, I entertained some doubts. In nursing school, they'd taught that such tremendous neglect as Heather had endured would cause irreparable damage.

Arriving home from work, my husband looked quite dapper, "Mr. Establishment," with his short dark hair, white shirt, navy-blue tie, and wingtip shoes. Jim worked as a computer programmer for the dental school, and his office was not too far from the PICU. Fourteen years earlier, we'd met at a rugby party. Back then he wore a cowboy hat atop his curly hair, an inside-out Mickey Mouse T-shirt, and scruffy tennis shoes. Back then he worked at a grocery store.

While preparing dinner, it seemed a good time to broach the topic of Heather with Jim. "Haven't you seen her when you check on Maria?" I asked. Jim knew her too, because she was often at our house. Jamie was friends with Maria's daughter, Jessica.

"So many sick kids, how would I know the child from the others?" Jim responded, sounding exasperated at my dreamy musings. Suppressed tension twitched a small muscle along his upper cheek. He smacked a heavy mug onto a bunch of garlic cloves and tossed the aromatic pulp into melting butter. I sliced a sweet onion, and thought on how I might lighten his resistance.

"Maybe if she comes to us as a foster child for a short while, we can recruit someone to adopt her," I suggested. My persistent talking backfired and added bricks to the wall growing between us.

No double older dreams figured into his hesitant thinking. With a gypsy-like spirit, we envisaged rambling around the North American continent in a van towing a pop-up camper. We longed to backpack trails in the Great Smoky Mountains, then venture farther west to observe buffalo grazing the prairie lands, and even farther to watch orcas breaching the waters off Seattle. Caring for such an ill child would surely squash such possibilities.

Later, standing on the front sidewalk, I gazed at the evening sky. In glowing splendor, the moon rose above the trees. Celeste slowed her car to a stop, and I jumped in. She made a left turn onto Archer Road, driving past a wooded trailer park. A mix of vehicles moved along the highway—agricultural flatbeds, sportsters, and pick-up trucks. Loops of rope tethered a double mattress to the hard-top of an aged Cadillac. Celeste accelerated and passed ahead lest the bed come loose and launch at us.

Arriving at the hospital, we parked, strode into the lobby, and obtained our visitor passes. Inside the PICU, silent Heather slept while the ventilator puffed life-sustaining breaths. Maria sat, keeping vigil next to Kyle's crib. Her hands flew, crocheting a blanket. Celeste asked a few haunting questions about his lethal congenital heart defect, then we initiated a happier conversation about nothing of importance. The trivial conversation dwindled. My concentration drifted to the voiceless child.

Heather was real, not some anonymous unfortunate in a newspaper article that was easy to pass over. What gifts lay hidden in this fragile baby, little bigger than a newborn and not much more alert? She couldn't even move her hands. Her head drooped. Emotion filtered my vision, blinding me to the drooling, the blue veins woven across her forehead, dusky skin, and misshapen skull, mattress-flattened from lying still too long.

"What medications is she on?" I asked her nurse.

"Some for her lungs. We hope one day she won't need the ventilator or trach tube."

"Anything else wrong with her?"

"Nothing," she said

"How would my husband and I become foster parents?"

"Hold on," she interrupted. "At long last they've found a prospective couple—they're coming next week."

Out of seemingly nowhere, sudden tears dampened my eyes.

She noticed. "Sorry," she said.

On the weekend, Jim wooed me in a sweet voice to go tubing down the Ichetucknee. The crystal clear river flowed at a constant spring-water temperature of 72 degrees. "Come on, it'll be fun," he insisted.

"It'll be chilly," I replied, and pantomimed being cold to make the kids giggle.

Inner-tube vendors popped up along the roadside. We stopped and loaded two large ones and a small inflatable boat. A trail padded with worn wood chips marked the way to the departure dock and three-hour float. Tall bald cypress trees lined the banks on both sides.

"Jump in, Mom!" Tony coached.

"It's freezing!" I protested.

"I'll help," Jim teased, jostling my shoulders as if to push me into the cold water, then he deftly cannonballed over my head, whooping in exhilaration as he bobbed back up through the river's surface.

Jamie climbed onto her tube, situating herself like a hovering starfish so that as little as possible of her bottom, arms, and legs touched the nippy water. I snapped the buckles on Tony's life jacket, and we crawled into the small inflatable boat.

The current carried us along. An occasional eddy bore us toward the shallows, swirling us in circles. Alligators claimed the territory as home. We'd never seen the stealthy reptile, but had floated past a swimming cottonmouth snake. Downstream, red-cheeked slider turtles sunned themselves on fallen logs.

Laughter pealed around the bend. On the shore, kids waited their turn to drop into a deep water hole. Jamie scrambled up the bank to join the Tarzan group.

"Is it too shallow? Are there rocks? I'm scared," Jamie quizzed one of the waiting boys.

"I made the rope swing," the boy bragged in reply. "Are you going or not? How old are you anyway? My pal is not frightened, and he's only in kindergarten," the boy taunted, then pushed ahead, caught hold of the sturdy knot and let fly. As he made his way back up the shore, he shouted encouragement to Jamie. "It's easy. Go, go, go!"

Jamie wrapped her arms around the rope, scrunched her eyes, and launched herself. In utter silence, she pierced the water like a falling arrow. The boys cheered.

Emerging from the chilly water, gooseflesh erupted all over her thin body.

Jim switched on the heat for the drive home. Hand-scrawled roadside signs advertised "Hot Boiled Peanuts." He slowed to park near to the big cauldron simmering over a wood fire. The cook ladled the steaming deliciousness into a couple of plastic bags insulated with brown paper sacks.

Briny, hot broth dripped down our chins, hands, and shirts. We used our teeth to crack the outer peanut shell. Our fingers pulled apart the loosened halves, and then we ate the inner soft and salty nuggets.

Jim resumed driving, and the kids dozed off.

At home, after baths and children in their pajamas, I mentioned the touchy topic of Heather. I thought Jim might be more amenable, if we were only back-up. "An already licensed foster family is coming to meet Heather. If they don't want her, she'll go to that horrid place." I wanted to call HRS (health and rehabilitative services) to find out the requirements.

"No inquiries," he directed, making clear that I better not cross that line.

"But doesn't she deserve a family?"

"It's hard enough providing for our two children," he countered.

"We'd make it work, same as we did with Tony. We went ahead and gambled that the baby and I would be okay, even when the doctor suggested ending the pregnancy."

Sweet Jamie was overcome by Heather's plight. Intrigued, Jamie and Tony scooted closer. "Please, Daddy, we'll be good; I'll do my chores," Jamie said.

"And I'll go to bed when you tell me," Tony promised. He knelt on the carpet and leaned in closer. "Please," Tony whispered into his father's ear.

I lingered with each of my children as I tucked them in. I began to shiver as I thought of Heather being condemned to an institution. What if Jim never changed his thinking?

CHAPTER 3] SMALL BABIES

In the morning, we took the kids to our favorite diner for breakfast. The young hostess seated us in a corner booth. Its table top was streaked wet from a cleaning rag. Tony tore open a sugar packet, then four more, drizzling the grains into his ice water.

"Honey, careful, the plate is hot," the waitress said as she served us plates laden with pancakes.

I tried to avoid thinking about Heather and instead appreciate my healthy family. Jamie rehashed her soccer game. Jim and I planned a weekend trip to my hometown for the next Shuttle launch. My father, Fritz Widick, worked on the early Atlas blow-ups to the successful Apollos that flew men to the moon. He was incredulous that a small-town Kansas boy ended up working for NASA as an aerospace engineer. We watched almost every launch from up close. Giant balls of fire thrust each rocket skyward. Thunderous undulations would shake the ground beneath our feet, fanning out and reaching observers more than thirty miles away.

An old man in a jockey cap smiled when he passed by on his way out of the diner. "Nice-mannered children," he said.

I dropped Jim and the kids at home, then ventured onward to the PICU.

When I arrived, a technician diverted me to the small waiting room because of visitation restrictions. I sat down on the floor near to Maria, drawing my knees up and hugging them close. No parents directly questioned the lock-out policy. An unshaven father stretched out on the carpet, using his arm as a pillow. Some simply accepted that they had no choice. Others feared complaints might affect a child's medical care.

Policy required parents to leave during invasive procedures, new admissions, and shift change. Staying overnight to comfort your ill child was prohibited. None were permitted in before noon so doctors could examine an ill child and write notes without interruption, which made asking questions difficult. Most information came secondhand, filtered through a nurse.

Research had disproved most of the policy's reasoning.

At long last the block-out ended. The technician beckoned us to form a line. The whole scene reminded me of a high-security prison. Yet the children's only "crime" was illness, and the families' was love.

Kyle slept in his crib. Maria crocheted, and I fiddled with a crossword puzzle. I glanced over at sickly Heather. Taped to her finger was a pea-sized monitor that glowed orange and monitored oxygen levels in her blood. It would sound an alarm to alert staff if her oxygen levels dropped.

Celeste soon joined us. Her expression became pensive as she watched a nurse loosen the oxygen mask covering Heather's trach, letting it dangle in front of the baby's chest. The nurse inserted a slender catheter through the small one's tracheotomy tube and applied suction. Heather's eyes opened, not focusing on anything, otherwise she made no response to the invasion of her body, no cough, nothing. Was Heather mentally not there or did she simply accept unpleasant sensations as normal?

"What are you doing?" Celeste asked the nurse.

"Her muscles are too weak to cough out secretions," the nurse explained. Suctioning removed mucous puddling in the tube. Dry spittle could form a plug and smother her. The poor baby suffered air hunger each time the scenario occurred.

"What is that?" Celeste asked, pointing to the constant positive airway pressure machine. Breathing effort is reduced by its infusing a steady flow of air to keep inflated tiny alveolar air sacs that would otherwise collapse.

"CPAP, we hope to wean her off it one day. Prior attempts, she's always tired." During weaning, trial sprints of self-breathing are lengthened until respiratory muscle strength and endurance increases to where a baby can sustain breathing without assistance.

Celeste peppered the nurse with more questions. "What's there to worry about with a tracheotomy?" Celeste asked, voice quiet and sincere.

"Many things. Worst is if the tube slips out. Soft tissues surrounding the opening in her neck would collapse, and she'd suffocate in minutes."

Celeste turned to me, her face both jovial and distressed, displaying a Celeste-only coy expression. "Convince Jim to let you guys bring her home. I'll be her favorite aunt," she said.

"Maybe I can," I answered.

No conversation followed, just an awkward, not peaceful silence. I headed upstairs to labor-and-delivery and went to work. I thought differently on the birth of the tiny babies. Might they suffer the same airway damage that Heather had?

Emergencies and premature babies were the daily routine at the busy, high-risk referral center, so busy that sometimes we walked eight miles in a single shift. Sometimes joyful and calm, but often nervous work. Before any birth, we took stock of resuscitative equipment and medications in the delivery room. First breaths require immense effort to rid the lungs of liquid and inhale air.

Right away I assisted with the birth of a preemie. I thought of Heather and the threshold of her life. The tiny baby's race against death started when he didn't cry and breathe as soon as he was born. Immature lungs were failing, and we had to intervene fast. The poor wee infant suffered the panic of asphyxia and a chill of evaporating fluids.

The obstetrician quickly placed the fragile baby, paper-thin skin, into the Ohio®—a crib equipped with oxygen, heaters, and bright lights.

Short, terse commands replaced all idle talk. We now existed as eyes and hands. Quick glances at our peers confirmed our silent thoughts; nimble fingers hurried to perform delicate tasks. We worked on, enclosed in a palpable sphere of tension.

A doctor intubated the little one's mouth and throat so a hand-squeezed air bag could pump in oxygen to lessen his distress. My turn again. I listened to his chest with a stethoscope, my index finger tapping out each beat of his heart in the air as a visual reference for members of the team.

"The rate is above one hundred," I called. "Breath sounds present in both lungs."

I felt the watching father's anguish for a split second before refocusing on the job at hand. With time thus suspended, I'd not know if seconds or hours were passing. A lifeline was swiftly slipped into the umbilical cord for drawing blood and giving medications. His limp body didn't respond, not yet. The bruises on his head would make me wince tomorrow but not today. A lot of preemies get them because there's no cushion of fat to protect them as they are squeezed through the birth canal.

Puff, puff, puff went the oxygen, and his cyanotic flesh blushed pink. He wiggled a hand and a foot and struggled to take a breath on his own. At last there was space for feeling, and we rejoiced at his spunk. The first round, and we had won.

With patches stuck on his chest to monitor vital signs and surgical gloves filled with warm water gently tucked beside his abdomen, our little one rested quietly in momentary calm before his mobile universe took off in a headlong rush to the neonatal intensive care unit.

Weighing in at three pounds, he'd fit in the palms of my hands; but he was a fighter. The monumental courage often seen in such a small scrap of life is incredible. Parents need it, too, when they hear the doctor's words: "If he survives the first three days, he ought to make it; but be prepared. Often a baby takes a turn for the worse before getting better."

CHAPTER 4] NO BOTTLES

The moment I'd met the child, she captured my heart. My thoughts changed to giving Heather a permanent forever home, not a temporary one. Either option required that Jim and I duplicate the equipment and medical care that the intensive care unit provided.

My husband freaked when I changed my pestering to the word *adoption*, though he probably knew that is what I meant all along. "Having a large family didn't include taking in other people's children," he said. Jim's father agreed it was folly, "You'll go broke."

My parents expressed a healthy skepticism. "If Heather comes to your home, and it's too tough, you can always give her back," my dad stated.

"But you haven't met her," I replied, leaving out select details.

A spattering of brown hair barely covered Heather's scalp. Her head was mattress-flattened from lying still too long. The corners of her mouth turned down in a perpetual pout, and she never moved her lips. Her skin had a bluish translucence.

Something happened that jarred my confidence, and I concluded that unsettling events might become the norm. A nurse unsnapped the faded terry sleeper to inspect and clean the smooth skin of Heather's belly below her left ribs. I gawked in disbelief at the blemish of a gastrostomy button—a plastic plug. Its far end was positioned inside her stomach. The nurse fit a thin feeding tubing into the plug's central opening and held aloft a dispenser. Deftly she poured a bottle of formula into the device and dripped in nutrition. Flowing by gravity, she lifted it higher to increase its speed.

The sight struck me like a lightning bolt; I'd never seen a tube-fed baby. I swallowed hard. Never had I given any thought as to what nourished Heather, and had failed to notice the lack of bottles.

"Can I hold the child while she's being fed?" I asked the nurse, trying to sound matter-of-fact.

"Who are you? Not just anybody can do her 'yummy,'" she asked, mellowing after accepting my bona fides.

Recollection of a paper that I'd read in nursing school prompted my request. A young mother who'd been tube-fed by a machine-fed apparatus for the first months of her life would not hold or cuddle her own infant during feedings. She propped the baby in an infant seat while sitting an arm's length away—not talking or displaying affection toward him. Researchers theorized that she'd learned the behavior because she was fed without any human contact.

After work and glad to be home, I padded down the hall and peeked in on my young son, curled up under his bedspread. Jim was stretched on the couch, watching television. "Had a good day," he said. When he told me about it, he began laughing so hard that he hugged his chest, and tears seeped from his eyes. "Tony dragged the old plastic baby bathtub outside, hoisted it on top of the picnic table, and pretended it was a boat. He climbed in, while holding his fishing rod, the one with a push-button reel. Determined to fish, he tied on a Lincoln log for bait and cast for the oak trees, for hours. He'd reel in, and the line would slip off the branches, never tangled.

"So I took him to Lake Geneva to catch real fish with gills. Better warn you though, Tony wants a dog," Jim said. "A golden lab would race down the dock and jump in, swim fast after whatever she spied. Loop back around, pause to play a little fetch the stick with Tony."

My sweet tooth begged indulgence. I dumped a box of brownie mix into a glass bowl and cracked the first egg, using both my hands.

"Show you something," Jim said, flashing a playful countenance. Grasping the second egg with a solitary hand, he tapped it, manipulated the shell with thumb and fingers in a swift motion, letting raw egg white and yolk slide into the batter.

"So clever," I complimented the master egg-cracker. I stirred the mixture. Batter dripped on my shirt when I sampled a mouthful. Jim wasn't interested in a spoonful.

"Tony and Jamie would want some," I said.

Before I could repress the question, words came tumbling out. "Have you thought any more about it? Somehow I know Heather is meant to become family."

Jim didn't answer.

Tense silence.

"Same as we did with Tony. If we adopt Heather, we'd accept the risks and roll with the outcomes. No kids come with a guarantee. Tony defied predictions; he turned out perfect."

Hoping to soften Jim's defensiveness, I got out some albums. There was a cute photo of Tony in his baptismal frock. Next picture was Father John Oliver pouring water over Tony's head from a carafe.

"Has Kyle been baptized?" Jim asked.

"I don't know."

We turned farther back to Jamie's baptism. Grandmother blamed Jim when at first the priest refused to bestow the sacrament.

Problem was that Jim and I no longer attended church each Sunday. We worked a lot of weekends.

"Why is an innocent baby penalized because her parents are rotten?" my dad teased. He turned serious. "How come it is so important?" He considered himself agnostic at the time.

"It just is," I answered.

"A white lie might resolve the issue," suggested my dad. "Tell Father Walsh that forever-more you'll attend weekly services."

"You can't fib to a priest," Jim balked at the idea.

Father Walsh, sounding quaint in his Irish brogue, suggested a compromise. "Confirm that you'll give serious consideration to regular attendance," he said. We assured him that we would. He baptized Jamie in the same church where he'd performed the ceremony for our marriage. Yet life got busier, and months often passed without Jim and me ever seeing an altar.

I reminded my husband that he said I could have plenty of children.

"And," he retorted, "after energetic Jamie was born, I said one was enough."

"You were being funny," I said.

"Heather is so very sick," he replied.

"The more reason to have the comfort of a family," I said. "Nursing skills I can teach you. Perseverance is channeled stubbornness, no problem there. Working opposite shifts would preclude the need to hire a specialized sitter for both of us to remain employed."

He didn't reply, so I continued. "Sometimes it's necessary to take a plunge, feet first, eyes closed, and hold your breath," I said softly. Perhaps he'd come to believe the saying was wisdom, not folly. Maybe he'd flip-flop his stance as he sometimes did, either to appease or other times to annoy. Sometimes over something as mundane as going out for ice cream, or major, like buying a house.

Despite Jim's objections, I figured he believed the opposite.

We'd persisted three years to have our son. I had a lot of problems carrying him. Heather was the very ill baby Tony could have been, the possibility we had feared.

Grandma Jean (Jim's mom) always tells the story the same way of that fateful Christmas day and my early pregnancy with Tony. "Almost dropped a whole sack of flour on the floor, it was as if a bomb detonated, all noise and commotion then silence." Grandma Jean was mixing dough for an apple pie crust when she'd answered the phone. I was the caller, and frightened. Earlier, I'd reluctantly left the family's festivities to work the evening shift. In a sudden twist, I'd gone from the role of nurse tending to women having babies to being the pregnant patient in the hospital bed.

Jim and I had already lost two pregnancies. With the previous one, I was hospitalized early on. Only the placenta was developing; the baby wasn't there. It was rapidly enlarging and had to be scraped out. With the other preceding pregnancy, I kept bleeding. The doctor put me on bedrest, but to no avail.

That Christmas day of the pie-making, I was four months pregnant. Inside my belly, the baby Tony, whom we then called "Twinkle" (for twinkle, twinkle, little star, how I wonder *who* you are), weighed about 4 ounces. My head hurt very badly. A co-worker checked my blood pressure. Way too high, so the doctor admitted me to the hospital. Without thinking, the obstetrician-in-training blurted out that for my well-being, she might terminate my pregnancy.

No way, I reeled. That won't be happening. If we were to lose the baby Twinkle, Jim and I would have ceased trying for a second child. It was too emotionally exhausting.

Luckily, my blood pressure normalized without any intervention other than keeping off my feet. My primary obstetrician prescribed no work and bedrest for the duration.

For the baby to survive, an additional 96 days inside my belly would create a very slim chance. Sustaining the pregnancy for 110 days would greatly increase the odds, and if my body cooperated, enduring a staggering 160 days of resting in bed to give birth to a fully mature baby.

Bedrest meant no income from me. Crisis as Jim had just resigned his long-houred management position with Publix Super Markets to study computer science at the community college. After graduation, Jim hoped to land an eight-to-five job. My parents insisted on subsidizing our budget for the six months I lay in bed, on the couch, or on a thick quilt on the grass in our back-yard.

When premature labor threatened, the dedicated obstetrician came to our home, instead of having me go to the office. Diligence paid off. Tony was born full-term and a plump eight pounds one ounce.

CHAPTER 5] DOZEN CALLS

A s I cut the brownies, I thought on how the fear that we'd lose Tony to a premature birth might be an additional shard that fueled my drive to assist Heather. I carried the brownie over to Tony and sat down on the couch. Jim interrupted my thoughts.

"Perhaps, are you going to the PICU tomorrow?" he asked.

"In the afternoon," I replied.

"I'll find you there," he said.

"To meet Heather?" I asked.

"Yes, all right, okay," he stammered.

"What changed?" I asked. He did not answer. Maybe he didn't know.

Jim entered the PICU, and I met him at the sink. We scrubbed our hands, utilizing the detailed wash technique of surgeons. "Heather has a cold virus and looks pitiful," I warned, as we walked to where she lay listless in her crib.

A kind woman holding a cloth bag approached us. "Are you the potential foster parents? I'm Sally, one of the nurse-specialists. I wash her soiled clothing and purchase her new outfits," she said and began removing garments from the bag.

We apprised her of our interest.

"We might still need you. Potential foster parents always renege. I'll tell the docs about you," Sally said. She wrote our names down, then shocked Jim by suggesting that he hold Heather.

"Go ahead, you'll do fine," I encouraged as he put on a cover gown.

Sally scooped Heather up, careful to not disturb all the monitor wires and ventilator tubing, and placed her in Jim's outstretched arms. He held the sickly child with a cautious sensitivity. Her feverish cheek was hot as a towel straight from the dryer, but she smelled of sickness rather than fresh laundry. She was limp as a ragdoll. Her eyes didn't focus. Perhaps she was blind, maybe deaf, maybe retarded.

The expression on Jim's face—I'd only seen twice before, when he first held our newborn daughter, and then our son. Using that mysterious, silent communication, Heather claimed Jim, same as she had me.

My husband linked my arm as we walked back to his office, both of us lost in our own private musings.

Breaking the silence, I said, "In case that couple declines, I'll find out how to become licensed as foster parents."

"Don't," Jim cautioned, his hand grip tightening on my forearm. "Wait and find out whether they decline." That was that. He was a yes or no man, and rarely expressed the thoughts behind his responses of few words. I'd respect his request and wait until he thought more on it.

Saturday morning breakfast, Jamie peeled the skin off some tangerines. Finicky, she picked the thick fibrous strands off each plump fruit. Tony pasted the stringy stuff under his nose like a mustache. He popped a juicy section into his mouth, swallowing all seeds.

Out front, the whirling tap of the jump rope slapped the concrete drive every few seconds. Jim could sustain the exertion twenty minutes and not get winded, while conversing with a friend the whole time. Perspiration glistened on his muscles and dampened his white T-shirt.

"Mark challenged me to a street competition," Jim said, as he walked into the house, followed by my good friend.

"It'll be amusing, come along," Celeste invited. She'd stopped by to show off their new jai alai equipment. Tony examined the tightly woven reeds of the throwing cesta. Jamie grabbed the bowl of tangerines, and we all followed them down the street, to Celeste and Mark's home, two houses down.

"Tommy Salami," Tony hailed his across-the-street buddy to tag along.

"Tony Baloney," Tom saluted. They gathered sticks and played fetch with the Hoffenberg's pet German shepherd.

"Baron is so fun. Can we have a puppy for Christmas?" Jamie asked.

"Tony proposed getting a dog the other day. I think you two are scheming," I replied, and then spoke more seriously. "Remember about that baby girl, Heather. If she comes to live with us, a pet would be risky; dog hair would get into her trach and lungs. One day, we'll get a puppy," I promised.

"Marky, I want a son as cute as Tony," Celeste said to her husband, initiating a flirtation. "Don't you want a chip off the old block for all the guy hobbies?"

"But he has me," Jim rebutted.

"Yeah, I have Jim," Mark replied, deadpan.

"Name the future son, Nicholas, then call him Nickle the Pickle so he can hang out with Tommy Salami and Tony Baloney." I giggled at my own stupid joke.

Celeste and I sat down on the curb for a better vantage to watch our handsome athletes.

Mark strapped the cesta to his hand, positioned the hard ball into its pocket, and threw it. Jim fired up his afterburners and surged to scoop the ball and propel it back. They powered several successful exchanges in a row, racing crisscross about the street and over the lawns.

Jim lunged low, missing a swift pass. Off-balance, he slung off his cesta and turned the awkward motion into a cartwheel. Cute improvisation, he pretended to stumble, and then spun around until plopping down with great flourish to sit right next to me. "Well, hello," he said, and threw his sweaty arm across my shoulders.

Celeste had deftly scooted out of his way to prevent getting sat upon. She startled us by getting serious. "I went to the PICU today," she stated. Abruptly she turned to gain Jim's attention, gazing at him with wide boring eyes, and spoke her message, directly to him, "Maria said Heather's prospective foster family never showed for their appointment."

I kept quiet, took a deep breath and slowly exhaled.

Jim's quick comment jettisoned unspoken emotion to the umpteen power. "Even though I said no to the pursuing adoption, I meant yes," he confessed.

"Were you struck by lightning?" I asked. Jim liked blunt comments; they amused him. "Or maybe playing jai alai cleared your thinking."

"Most would label such a declaration—crazy talk," Celeste said, soft laugh lines crinkling her face.

"What changed your mind?" I asked.

"Heather deserves a family, and we are it, simple as that," Jim answered. The concept was only simple if steeped with faith. Let fear simmer in, then better descriptors would be mindboggling, overwhelming, too many scary unknowns and even scarier facts. A forever trach meant it would be forever impossible for her to swim and snorkel. Most summers, we vacationed in the Florida Keys.

The next day, Jim and I again visited the PICU together. A vigorous toddler ran to him and showed off his tiny black race car. The boy waved at a passing nurse, who came and squatted down beside him, letting him hop aboard her back. A broad smile illumined his face as he bounced along on a piggyback ride.

Alexander's inaudible laughter suited the unit's somber atmosphere, though inconsistent with his exuberant demeanor. Like Heather, the boy had a trach tube protruding from his neck; and had never lived anywhere but the hospital. Nurses doted on him, and his bedside was piled high with toys and picture books. He responded to the attention with glee. Unlike Heather, who seemed a sleeping caterpillar within an invisible cocoon.

A male nurse had mentioned the boy. He and his wife planned to bring the youngster home as a foster child and eventually adopt him. In three weeks the two-year-old would bid the PICU good-bye, for the first time in his life.

On an informational display board, an HRS flyer begged for couples to foster parent several hospitalized, medically needy children. Eager for guidance, we paged the hospital social worker and asked her about it.

"Out of county caseworkers suggested posting that. Though the kids are in the hospital here, they are assigned to the HRS department in the county where their mother resides. But I can't help; records are confidential. Besides, we might have a placement," she said. "Oh, I just love Heather," she gushed.

"Do you know which county Heather's mom lives in?" I asked.

"I can't tell you," she murmured.

Curiosity had me review the hand-written delivery log book until I found the day of Heather's birth. No addresses were listed, but it detailed time of delivery, Apgar score, baby's weight, complications, and attending doctors and nurses. There was my name. I shivered. I was one of the nurses who tended to Heather's birth. I remembered much about the night.

That evening had unfolded quite strangely. A small hospital was sending us a patient who'd gone into labor ten weeks early. Even riskier, the baby was lying sideways in the womb instead of head first. When the birth sac ruptured, unimpeded amniotic fluid would gush out past the baby, and carry along a loop of umbilical cord. Ensuing contractions would trap the loop of pulsing lifeline between the baby and the mother's pelvic bones, squeezing off the baby's vital supply of oxygen. Death ensues in minutes.

Our charge nurse assigned me to assess the transfer patient upon her arrival. If feasible, we'd administer medication to stop her contractions. Otherwise emergency surgery would proceed rapidly. Until then, my job was to float and do tasks which I could immediately abandon.

All evening, we were crazy busy. The charge nurse insisted I remain actively waiting. In four years, that had never happened. Nine babies were born; two by cesarean section, almost a record. Near end of shift change, the transfer patient reached us on a stretcher. Blood dripped onto the floor from the sheets beneath her bottom. The quantity meant the mother and the baby in her womb were at risk for imminent death from massive exsanguination. Placental abruption had occurred. The afterbirth had partially separated and was bleeding between itself and the uterus. Some accumulating blood remained trapped, and some was leaking out through the birth canal.

Gail, a co-worker, and I intercepted the transport crew. In the main hallway, without moving the woman to the privacy of a room, we prepared her for surgery. Gail scrubbed the woman's laboring abdomen with antiseptic, while I inserted a Foley catheter to drain the bladder and keep it out of the way of the surgeon's knife. We rushed the woman into the operating room.

On-coming nurses assisted the anesthesiologist and obstetrician in preparation for the emergency cesarean section. Gail turned on the radiant heater and overhead lights of the Ohio® medical crib. I tested and arranged the resuscitative equipment and meds on a nearby table in anticipation of the likely scenario: a limp baby who failed to breathe.

The instant the obstetrician incised the uterus, an assistant suctioned bloody amniotic fluid into a collection container. The OB's skilled hands grasped the baby inside the woman's womb and guided the fragile premature baby head-first into the world. The tiny babe breathed as the doctor handed her over. My friend and I positioned the wee infant in the Ohio®, monitoring her efforts to live. Gently, we dried her with a warmed blanket. On-coming nurses took over and transported the three pound baby in the mobile medical crib to the neonatal intensive-care unit. She was bound to tucker out.

Wow! Heather was that same baby girl. Destiny chose me to be her mother, I hoped.

Fear that Heather would end up in an institution continued to gnaw at me. To make Tony content long enough to make some inquiries, I dumped out a bucket of wooden blocks. Nearby I placed a plate of cookies. I settled down on my bed and dialed Alachua County's foster-care unit, only to be shuttled through various unhelpful employees. The same thing happened with adoptions.

"Don't you know the goal of foster care is reunification with the family?" the last one snarled. What family? I pondered, wanting to growl back. I considered calling Alex's soon-to-be dad, but didn't know his last name. Remembering he'd mentioned a foster parent association, I tried them, and an informative lady answered.

"Hang in there," she encouraged. "If you can't persevere, you have no business parenting difficult kids." She shared some insights about HRS and provided a new contact, whom I hoped would be synonymous with Lady Luck.

With renewed optimism, "Linda Taylor, please," I said and repeated my story.

"Heather's not in our computer," she said.

"If it makes a difference, both the mom and tentative foster family live outside of Alachua County," I said.

"Even so, if a placement had been made, I'd know," Linda Taylor said, but offered no direction.

No placement—maybe it was a possibility, this fantastical idea of Heather coming to our home. To think I believed a single call would be enough, that they'd be thrilled that we wished to become Heather's parents. Attending a series of classes, fingerprints, background checks, and an investigation as to our character were requisite. How could we initiate that process?

Mentioning foster care and adoption in the same sentence was tricky. The goal of foster care was reunification with the parents; the goal of adoptions was a permanent, forever home. Which created a dilemma, as Heather needed both. HRS formal proceedings had a certain order, creating the proverbial Catch-22. If guidelines were followed literally, without flexing, instead of their essence, her timeline and our timeline might not mesh.

Good fortune visited; I ran into the male nurse who had told me about the flyer. He named off some districts that were recruiting foster parents.

Armed with new information, I rang Park County.

"She isn't in our division," stated the supervisor.

"Can you please double-check? I think she is," I countered.

"Well, let me see." She put me on eternal hold before uttering her answer. "We do have her case, but we've already found a home."

"Remember us, if something goes awry," I replied, and thanked her for the assistance.

So many children needing homes, yet only dead-ends. I took to the street for a soul-easing hen session with the neighbors. A good night's sleep didn't quiet my mind, so in the morning I phoned Linda Taylor. "She's not in, but you can talk to Debbie." Oh, goose, more runaround! But I was wrong.

"Wouldn't it be ideal for Heather to be placed with foster parents who want to adopt her?" I asked. Heather's case would soon shift from the foster care unit to adoptions. To my astonishment, she agreed.

"If someone requests priority processing for both foster parenting and adoptions, we can do it. The foster parent course starts Tuesday. Applications are given to those who show up. Please attend." Debbie's words were as refreshing as an ocean breeze blowing through a hot summer cabin.

Yet the island of peace was fleeting. I perceived doubt the minute Jim got home. He'd stopped by the PICU. "We don't need to go Tuesday," he announced.

"Why?"

"Heather's not going to an institution. That foster family came, and they want her."

"I'm not convinced," I said.

"They won't risk banking on unlicensed us, if they have a licensed family." Jim spoke softly, laying out the dilemma. "They don't know whether we're just talk, no substance."

"You're correct," I said, slumping into a chair. "But what if the others still back out, then she'll go to that awful place. Can't we attend classes?"

"All right, all right," he conceded.

I reached for my guitar and began strumming the chords for the Beatles' "Let It Be," singing its simple words of comfort and faith.

Tuesday seemed endless in spite of efforts to keep busy. I cleaned house. Tony took a long nap. Jim got home. He loosened the knot on his tie and hung it in our closet. Pepperoni pizza cooled on a wooden cutting board. Seated on a braided rug, Jamie and Tony lounged in their pajamas, playing a card game with their baby-sitter.

Jim and I departed for the HRS licensing course and its unexplored new territory.

Eight couples took a seat around an oblong table. Debbie's sunny disposition got us talking, sharing stories and fears. One seasoned family had already adopted a difficult child and sought to provide shelter to his younger brother. Another couple aspired to helping troubled teenagers.

The next man spoke with anguish. "My stepfather beat me," he said, his whole body quivering. "No child should go through that. They might not let me be a foster dad, but I'll stick with the whole course."

"We want to aid a hospitalized little girl," Jim said when our turn came, careful not to mention adoption.

Debbie spelled it out in simple words, her brief statement sobering. "These kids are all handicapped. They have been abandoned, neglected, and physically or sexually abused," she said. "They have health or behavioral problems, serious ones. They are not sweet little cherubs, and may harm your children, forcing the agonizing decision to return them." More sobering lecture followed.

"Though we hope to reunite families, in some cases we recommend terminating parental rights. Other times parents voluntarily relinquish them."

Perhaps none of the statistics on troubled children applied to Heather, as she had medical problems. Hmmm. Neglect, extreme psychosocial deprivation; check yes. She fit that category. Heather languished in a hospital. Physical abuse, check yes—surgery and tubes are very painful. No purposeful movement. Maybe deaf, blind, and severely retarded. Never loved. Unable to love? The last possibility would be the hardest to swallow.

To us, predictions were irrelevant. We believed Heather had potential and that fate destined us to become her parents. Was there such a match for each waiting child?

At the close of class, Debbie ran out of applications. She suggested meeting at her office the following morning.

We did. She gave me a brief tour, handed me the foster-parent application, then had me follow her down the hall to adoptions. The voice I heard through the doorway was the snarly one I'd encountered on the telephone.

"This is Mrs. Lurdan, the adoptions supervisor," Debbie said. We exchanged a few pleasantries, and Debbie summed up Heather's situation.

Without preamble, Mrs. Lurdan let the ax fall. "About the adoption application packet, I'm not giving it to you." She proferred no reason. Dumbfounded, I hurried out without asking, afraid I'd start weeping. If the process continued to get blocked, Jim and I had zero chance of becoming Heather's parents.

CHAPTER 6] NIGHT CLASSES

Maybe adopting Heather was more far-fetched than landing on the moon, and the dream of her growing up healthy, even loftier. But to sustain me, Man did indeed walk on the moon. I grew up watching every launch. Initially the rockets all blew up, and then majesty. Nothing is impossible.

"I don't understand," I grumbled to Celeste.

"Grade-school bullies don't disappear. They grow up," she said.

"Know any good lawyers?" I asked.

"Bobby might," she answered. He practiced real-estate law. In college Celeste worked at a drugstore he owned, now closed. She held him in high esteem, so much so, that when Mark and Celeste married, Bobby escorted her down the aisle as her father would have if still living. For twenty years they'd all been friends.

I worried Bobby might have no one to suggest. Impatient and thinking the more guidance the better, I phoned a lawyer who had done adoption work for a neighbor's family.

"A white baby girl," the attorney said. "They are in demand."

"Not one as sick as Heather," I answered.

"I have many clients wanting to adopt," he disagreed. His enthusiasm alarmed me. I felt nauseated and at the risk of sounding paranoid, I closed the conversation and dutifully waited for Bobby's advice.

A couple of days passed before Celeste conferred with me. Bobby recommended two attorneys. Both did a lot of work in juvenile court, and both were skilled at making crucial contacts. Women dominate the machinery of HRS, so Jim and I scheduled an appointment with the female attorney, Martha Lott.

Perhaps an attorney would know how to break the gridlock. The hospital social worker never contacted HRS to speed up our foster and adoption licensing process. "Too bad you didn't come around sooner. The Wilsons are experienced foster parents for medically-needy children," she'd said. Mrs. Wilson worked part-time, was five months pregnant, and already had four children— one of whom was disabled. She and her husband had agreed to keep Heather until the institution bed opened up.

"Excuse me. We'll keep visiting Heather—if that's okay?" I asked the social worker.

"It would be better if you didn't," she said. "The foster family will be getting acquainted."

I smiled, a fake one, a required one to make things turn out right; smiling not at her, but with the unknown that propelled me on this sane but insane quest.

Maria told me no one ever visited Heather. The foster parents wouldn't. No way would they have time. Some staff professed great affection, but never acknowledged Heather in any way when near.

Maybe it was splitting a gnat's hair, but the social worker had not specifically forbidden my visiting. Existing in a seemingly invisible and impenetrable cocoon, Heather's solitude was a concern if she actually became our daughter. With that in mind, each night once Jim arrived home, I'd go to the hospital. First stop was the main lobby desk. Though it had been tempting to give my friend's name, I always requested a pass to go to the PICU to visit Heather.

"That doesn't sound familiar. Is she a new admission?" the receptionist inquired. I shook my head negative. "Maybe you have the wrong unit?" she asked, continuing to search the patient roster. Heather had been hospitalized for more than fourteen months, the clerk's recognition of her name should have instantly clicked. Dismayed, I clutched my purse tighter. "She's in the first pod," I volunteered.

The receptionist surveyed the list once more, then handed over a pass with Heather's name on it. I rode the elevator to the second floor. Heather's nurse smiled when she saw me.

Evenings brought an illusion of quiet to the PICU. The hectic daytime pace of baths, tests, surgeries, doctor and student rounds was over. Yet emergency admissions and medical crises often disrupted the silence and sent the adrenalin of a spread-too-thin staff surging.

My tremulous approach to Heather's crib contrasted with the stark confidence of white walls and spotless floors. Vents blew cool air laced with the odor of cleaning products, not the pungent smells of illness. Heather reclined in an infant seat that was set inside her crib. She looked like a baby doll that had been tinted blue instead of pink. Struggling breaths heaved her small chest.

I picked her up, making sure to maintain the connection between her trach and the breath-blowing CPAP machine. I cuddled her close, keeping the rocker moving in an easy, lulling motion.

I didn't speak, just held her in a silent envelope of love. Her eyes acknowledged my face for a fleeting moment, about as quick as a single flutter of a hummingbird's wings. Without teeth, she had a peculiar habit of sucking her lips into her mouth like a toothless old woman. Saliva often pooled under her tongue and spilled down her chin.

Maria had already left for the day. Her baby slept. His heart raced near two hundred beats per minute.

Each evening I returned, murmuring soft words and introducing simple games. "Nose," I said and touched hers. I wiggled her toes and sang "this little piggy went to market." I read bedtime stories and never left until she fell back asleep. Then I'd gently tuck her in and check that all the alarms were working.

Alexander's bon voyage happened that same week. The night before, his new family slept over in a special PICU guest-room in case questions arose as they managed his care. All celebrated the monumental event in grand style with helium balloons, cake, and gifts. Except for the trach protruding from his neck, he appeared a robust and typical two-year-old when he walked out of the hospital for the first time ever, hugging a Raggedy Andy doll and sipping soda from a can. His new brother, a few months younger, toddled close behind. Surprisingly, Alexander's departure proved a boon for Heather. His doting nurses increased the time they spent with her.

Scare-you-out-of-your-wits night. That's what they called our third class. A panel of experienced foster parents and social workers tried to squash any soft, starry-eyed, do-gooder images we might hold by searing us with molten reality. It seemed they had combined the horrible transgressions of all foster kids and attributed them to one monster child, whom they implied was a typical foster kid at his best. Harsh tales sounded overstated, but most graduates complained that they weren't graphic enough.

"If tempted to redecorate your house or to buy new furnishings—don't!" a social worker cautioned. "These children are angry and get destructive; they may start fires or shred your furniture. Hide your knives and matches. Lock up guns and ammunition in separate cabinets. Suicide is a possibility at any age." She reemphasized the passionate warnings many times.

"'Oh, have I got a cute one for you!' Be careful when you're told that," a feisty middle-aged woman warned. "My kids are cute all right." She held up a picture. "See, they're gorgeous!" She laughed that fanatical way some giggle when things are too awful to cry.

"Prepare neighbors and friends for odd behaviors," a polite middle-aged man suggested. "Intolerant acquaintances may manipulate the system and falsely report foster parents as abusers to get foster kids thrown out of a neighborhood."

Coffee break brought a welcome respite. Jim was glad that most of the parental abuses didn't seem to apply to Heather, as she'd never lived with a parent.

Stark real-life statements from a heavy-set social worker opened the second half of the session. "Even in a good, long-term placement, removing a child from his biologic family is a serious form of abuse," said the man. "It may cause infinitely greater harm than what the parents are alleged to have done. Removal causes loss of one's culture, value clash and confusion, and to survive—a forced acceptance of a foreign one."

For the duration of class the heavy-set social worker delved into the traumatic stages a removed child traverses.

Shock numbs the child for the first few weeks, and he tries hard to please. Abruptly that ends when he opens his eyes and takes wavering steps toward absorbing his situation—he has lost his home, family, grandparents, aunts, uncles, cousins, friends, religion and place of worship, his school, pets, clothes, and toys. He is living with strangers who are very different. Rage floods his being, and he expresses it through destruction.

"Many kids get kicked out at this point. They may lose a dozen foster placements in one year," he said. "Licensed homes are scarce.

Each move among foster homes often means enrollment in a different school, rendering academic success and friendships almost impossible." Bounced-about foster children may live in as many as thirty-five different homes. Not all homes are safe. Instead of the idealistic wished-for havens, some foster parents victimize kids through emotional neglect or actual physical, mental, and sexual abuse.

A friend of mine grew up in an orphanage and thinks that option is better. She had stability in the roof over her head, always attended the same school, and lived with a familiar group of children even if members of the adult staff moved on. I was determined to provide Heather with the best option of all: a loving, stable family.

The belief that Jim and I were destined to parent Heather moved us onward, and we never pondered why. We hoped that the attorney, Martha Lott, might be a beacon guiding us through the darkness. In preparation for our meeting, Jim and I had ironed our clothes. Air conditioning blew cold in our decade-old Mercury Marquis. Cloudy skies dropped a quick, heavy rain, but the sun reappeared. Steamy vapor drifted off the pavement and hung suspended without a breeze to nudge it along.

Jim turned off a congested main street that was bordered with fast-food restaurants to take the scenic brick-paved route to downtown. Heritage oaks draped with Spanish moss shaded turn-of-the-century Victorian homes. A few blocks away, blistering concrete surrounded the modern courthouse, library, and city bus terminal.

In my purse I carried a small, important journal where I'd logged all our questions, jotted down events arranged into a time line, and scribbled notes about important conversations complete with date, hour, name, title, and intuitive impressions.

Jim locked the vehicle and strode alongside me in an energetic strut. He tossed the car keys skyward like a stringless, upward-thrust yo-yo. Eyes twinkling, jovial, he leapt to catch them, lest they drop to the ground. He gripped my hand and guided me as we quietly climbed the steps to the attorney's office. A secretary ushered us in to the consultation room. Martha Lott wore her hair loosely wound in a graceful twist and carried herself with poise.

We plunged right in and poured out our tale, using the journal as a guide, attempting to sound rational and calm. The palms of my hands dampened.

"How should we address you?" Jim asked.

"You are entrusting me with a highly personal matter, so please call me Martha," she said in a warm, confident voice. "If the mother still had custody, this would be easy. Since the state has declared Heather a dependent of the state, her mom has no say. HRS rules dictate all proceedings."

"How come it is so difficult?" I asked.

"Power," she said. "Some people like to control; others are lazy. The system is flawed, but it's all we have." She wrote swift words on her legal pad. "Our job is not to fix HRS. We accept the flaws and navigate through the imperfections for Heather's well-being."

"We brought this," Jim said, handing her a copy of the foster-care application—thirty pages of answers to questions about how we each grew up, family, marriage, discipline beliefs, finances, and friends. It contained employment references; questionnaires our two children filled out; and required handwritten welcome-to-our-home letters, one from each of us: Jim, Jamie, Tony, and me.

"I'll read it cover-to-cover before making any inquiries. I have to know all about you," Martha teased in an over-dramatic yet serious manner before easing into a smile. "What is pending?" she asked.

"An inspector is scheduled to scrutinize our home for fire hazards and general safety. Our fingerprints and background checks have already cleared," Jim answered.

"As soon as I know something, I'll get in touch. Nice to meet you," she said, escorting us out.

Later that afternoon, when I answered the phone and heard Martha Lott's voice, I whispered a prayer.

"Good news!" she exclaimed, "Diane Morris, the Park County foster-care supervisor, thinks you and Jim wanting to adopt is terrific, especially since you are a nurse. Plan is for Heather to initially leave the hospital with the other foster family, but she'll designate you and Jim as respite foster parents."

"So fast and fabulously encouraging. Thanks!" I said.

"One problem," Martha said. "There's no legal way to require visits. I told Diane I was worried about you and Jim losing your bond. She's all for frequent visitation, but you'll have to negotiate the arrangements."

"I'll introduce myself to the Wilsons," I said.

"When is her PICU discharge date?" Martha asked.

"Tentatively November 4, but first she has to undergo a bronchoscopy."

"Explain in more detail please," she said.

"Each month the surgeon examines Heather's trachea with a bronchoscope and inserts rods of increasing diameters in an attempt to stretch open the scarring of her airway," I said.

"A few concerns," she said, "find out whether your house wiring is adequate for her medical equipment and the CPAP breathing machine, and the cost of a back-up generator. It may be required in case a thunderstorm knocks out your electric power. Keep me apprised of what you find out."

"The nurses remove the CPAP when bathing her in the sink. Perhaps she'll be done with it," I said and we ended the conversation.

Previous weaning attempts ended with near bouts with death. Heather always tired, until her breathing ceased. Resumption of continuous CPAP and supplemental oxygen followed each failure. Stories of such bouts of hypoxia tweaked my momentary contemplation that predictions of extensive brain damage might hold credence.

Jim and I embraced a blind belief in the incredible resilience of the human spirit. I flipped the message of the theories that proposed that deprivation in early childhood doomed a child for emotional dysfunction and reduced intelligence. I'd heed the warning and take time to teach this little girl what she had missed. Each evening when I went to Heather, I rocked and cuddled and whispered tender lullabies. A momentous night rolled around.

I blinked at Heather.

She blinked back.

Coincidence?

I blinked again, and she blinked back, with no other change of her expression. All my countenance rejoiced at such a surprising and incredulous first communication.

We got a break. Postponement of Heather's bronchoscopy pushed back her potential discharge until November 17. I updated Martha Lott. "When do you finish classes?" she asked.

"The first week of November."

"There's a chance that Heather could go with you and Jim. Apprise me the minute your foster-parent license is one-hundred percent approved." Her encouragement and precise guidance let us think that, maybe, just maybe, our life would change in ways never imagined.

CHAPTER 7] LEGACY

For a needed break, we drove to my parents' home for the weekend. Heavy traffic slowed our progress through Orlando. Flashy billboards beckoned tourists to the Magic Kingdom. In the days before Disney, rows upon rows of splendid emerald-green trees laden with orange and yellow fruit covered the gentle hills. A few orchards remain. Each spring the sweet fragrance of citrus blossoms drifts everywhere."Mom, look!" Tony pointed at a quickly slowing jet, flying overhead, descending to land at the Orlando International Airport. It served as a sentinel heralding the last thirty-five mile stretch. The Beachline expressway traverses native Florida terrain—peat bog and swamp that are home to smallish deer, long-legged egrets stalking the river bank, drifting alligators, and mosquitoes swarming the scrub brush.

"Hold your breath until we reach the other side. Bet you can't," Jamie challenged as we drove over the tall bridge spanning the Indian River. Tony gulped a breath and pinched his nose. Jim opened a window, letting salty freshness breeze through. Sometimes it reeked of rotting sea grasses and dead fish. Looking north, we caught a glimpse of Kennedy Space Center. Around the bend lay Port Canaveral with its shrimp trawlers, scallop boats, and cruise-line ships.

"Only fifteen more minutes," I said.

"We're here!" Jim announced as he opened the door to my childhood home. Warm hugs and the aroma of chicken and fresh-baked bread greeted us. At dinner we caught up on the latest family happenings, and talk turned to Heather. I bragged about her determination to stay alive, her eyes that were no longer shrouded, but blinked with quiet enthusiasm.

"Who are her people?" queried my uncle.

"Perhaps Heather has suffered serious brain damage?" Dad asked.

"We think she has potential," Jim said, unsure how else to answer.

"Heather deserves a chance." I tried to explain our reasoning.

"What if she never talks? Is always confined to a wheelchair? You've seen some of those children." Their doubts persisted.

"Biological children don't come with guarantees," Jim asserted, making it clear the conversation was over. So did I, by excusing myself to assist in the kitchen.

I pondered the irony of the situation. As a teenager, I'd contemplated that if

I was never capable of becoming pregnant, I would want to adopt the perfect baby. I had held the same quandaries as they now did: theoretical concerns about whether a relinquishing biological mom might have used drugs or alcohol? Or did insanity run in the biological family?

The Atlantic Ocean was a little over a mile away.

Late afternoon is cooler and most pleasant at the beach. The ocean, always a constant friend, in all her moods erases unrest and imbues a sense of peace. Jim and I strolled arm-in-arm, barefoot, enjoying the feel of wet sand between our toes. Our rambunctious youngsters waded ankle-deep and skipped shells over the gentle waves that broke with a hiss of bubbling foam. It got later, and still we stayed. Twinkling stars and a rising moon glinted off the ocean, creating a sparkling reflection.

In bed that night the words of my relatives, like slivers of broken glass pricking my resolve, awakened me from a fitful sleep. My eyes wide open, yet fatigued; weighted down with thoughts of the unknown, I rolled toward Jim and placed my arm over his warm shoulder. Calmed by the sureness of him, I drifted into a peaceful slumber.

In the morning the whole clan hastened back to the beach. We quick-stepped over hot wooden decking that spanned dunes, abloom with yellow and purple flowers, and ran across scorching sand to the cool, damp tide line. Plunking down the gear, our children and their young cousins raced into the shallows.

At a distance the beach appears a uniform, boring beige. On closer inspection kaleidoscopic patterns emerge. Flowing water creates intricate ripple patterns and embellishes them with rainbow-colored periwinkle shells, squirmy, thumbnail-sized sand fleas, and tiny minnows. Bird tracks and footprints add their temporary stamp, and sand castles boast varying stages of glory. As we basked in the sun, the relatives turned talk once again to Heather.

"You'll go broke."

"What if she dies?"

"If she makes it to her fourth birthday, she's supposed to live," I responded.

"Has she been tested for AIDS?"

They didn't understand, and their mental vision didn't at all match the one Jim and I held, though theirs was probably closer to reality.

"Mike says to go for it. He thinks it's great," I said. Mike is my youngest brother.

"He is young," the skeptic replied.

"But he is a medical student and actually met her on his rotation through the PICU," I said.

"If she proves a burden, you could always give her back," an uncle said.

"You don't return family," Jim said quietly, repressing all emotions. Otherwise his words would have erupted with fury. Jim grabbed his red surfboard and paddled out, riding a wave in on his second try. Never me; I always wiped-out. Body surfing is my style. Push off with my feet, thrust my arms forward, and raw energy jettisons me into a tunnel of rushing water that shoots me along, maneuvering to avoid violent curls that can pitch my body with great force onto the scratchy seafloor.

Cowabunga!" hollered the kids, and we scrambled to submerge below a powerful on-coming wave. Pelicans dive bombed, making huge splashes as they scooped up the ocean's bounty.

After a while we all headed back to my parents' home. Relaxing by the pool, Dad fired up the grill and flipped thick burgers to sizzling. Exact same delicious ones he'd cooked for the Apollo astronauts before each launch. Crew and back-up crew knew Dad well. For the moon landings, he was chief test conductor for the lunar module. Jim encouraged my father to share a few stories from his career. Jamie and Tony climbed out of the pool and dried off with a towel.

"Tell the one about the Atlas, when the countdown was in progress," I suggested. The rocket stood ready, tethered to the launch tower, fully loaded with fuel. Scaffolding supported a circular platform around its perimeter. My dad and the key mission specialists walked along the platform, inspecting many things, including the thrust chamber.

"No one noticed a spraying pin-hole leak, except my clothing which was newly stained with a fine line of green lithium hydroxide. I needed something to stem its escape," Dad said. His face crinkled with increasing amusement at his ingenious quick fix. "Let me have that," Dad said to a gum-chewer. The Rocketdyne engineer handed over his chewed Dentyne, and Dad stuffed the wad into the hole. "All conferred and felt certain the patch would hold until launch." Dad explained, "At ignition, lithium hydroxide is fully consumed. It combines with oxygen and dampens the drumming forces of the starting explosions. We saved the taxpayers millions of dollars. That was in my younger days, I wouldn't do that now."

After dinner and baths, while Jim and I were playing cards with my parents, a phone call came from Maria with bad news about her little baby boy. "Annie," she sputtered. "Kyle is dying. The doctor is talking about a ventilator."

At about midnight, we pulled into the hospital parking lot. Words I'd often spoken to the parents of dying infants, now gave me counsel: Study your baby and latch on to one detail. It gives you something concrete to hold so you can release the dream.

Kyle lay in the Ohio®, his eyes closed, his face peaceful. Silently I prayed, sensing something different. I bundled him up and held him close, his weakening heart pulsing against my shoulder. His tiny being whispered, *my travail is over; it's okay.* I relieved Jim's watch over our sleeping children so he could spend some moments with Kyle.

Jessica came home with us. Jim inflated air mattresses and spread out sleeping bags. Tony curled up beside them. At 7:00 a.m. Bill phoned us. "I'm coming for my daughter," he said. "Kyle didn't make it."

Jim and I lingered in the foyer of the church, not wanting to enter. Rays of sunshine splintered through its stained-glass windows, igniting a portrayal of the flame of the Holy Spirit. Friends and family streamed in for Kyle's funeral. Everyone dressed in their Sunday best. Tony was young enough not to complain about his bow tie.

A simple sculpture of Mary adorned the basin of holy water with which we blessed ourselves. Jamie made the sign of the cross perfectly. Jim's strong hand guided Tony's. We filed into a pew near the front; and Celeste, Mark, and Haley dropped into the one behind. The rhythm of prayers and traditions of the Mass consoled us in our sorrow. Garbed in a white chasuble, the priest offered words of enduring wisdom and comfort. I draped my arms around Jamie and Tony and snugged them close. They rested their heads against me, and Jim slipped his arm across all of us.

Thoughts of Heather's mother and her loss flickered. I had caught my breath and stared when a tall woman appeared at Heather's cribside a month ago, bearing cookies and a juice bottle. Kyle was asleep in my lap, and I almost tipped over the rocker.

"Don't give her those!" a nurse admonished.

"She doesn't eat?" The tall woman's brow furrowed; her hand trembled as she placed the tokens of nourishment on the bedside table. Thin, about my age, and stiff with caution, she paced a circle away and then back to her daughter. She lifted Heather, rigid-armed, unaware of my presence, and held her near her chest.

I pondered rumors I'd heard and realized we'd never know the truth. She patted Heather's back mechanically. For a fleeting moment, she looked at her daughter warmly then gazed off, detached. At least I could share something good with Heather when she was older: I'd seen love in her mama's eyes—and overwhelming fear. After she left, the nurses gossiped among themselves.

"She relinquished Heather voluntarily because she couldn't handle the medical problems," muttered one.

"You can count the number of times that she's visited her daughter using the fingers of only one hand," grumbled another.

I reflected on the sorrows of both mothers and their contrasting griefs. The priest's intonations lulled me back to the present. "The Mass is ended; go in peace to love and serve the Lord." Some of the mourners left the church quickly while others lingered. Celeste again sank to her knees, shoulders shuddering with sorrow. Mark sat quietly next to her with his head bowed. In silent prayer I asked for guidance as tears flowed down my cheeks. Jim and I were among the last to offer condolences.

Kyle's death intensified our hope to give Heather a chance at life.

Navigating the system for Heather to possibly become our forever daughter felt like traversing on a high wire without having practiced, nor a safety net below.

On a brighter side, Heather chalked up daily progress. The doctors weaned her off the CPAP. No longer limited by a length of tubing connected to the breathing machine, the nurses carried her about, bestowing playful attention. Propped in a baby walker, she'd struggled to briefly hold her head erect. Elation showed in the wrinkle of her nose. She pushed her feet and accidentally scooted the walker a few inches. Her clumsy fingers still couldn't grasp anything. Drool spilled from her mouth. I chose only to see cocooned determination and brightening eyes that she blinked at me in greeting.

Jim and I completed the series of evening foster-care classes. Next hurdle for licensing was the social worker observing our family in our home on two different occasions. More delay, more patience; openings in her schedule were scarce. Debbie would question each of us, including the kids, in individual interviews.

"I hear you'll inquire about our sexuality?" I'd asked, steeling myself for that foray into our privacy.

"Just whether it's satisfactory," Debbie chirped. "Some tell more than I want," she added.

Even when fully completed, our HRS file would likely gather dust for untold days in a massive stack of papers awaiting an administrative stamp of approval. Unless an unforeseen circumstance pushed someone to request that we become a priority, we were status quo. Further narrowing any prospect of Heather leaving the hospital with Jim and me, the fire and safety inspectors postponed their scrutiny of our home.

In counsel our attorney reminded us to navigate the imperfect system and make it work for Heather. We stumbled forward, always trying to keep wedged open a chance of becoming Heather's permanent parents.

CHAPTER 8] NEEDED CONNECTION

On November 17, I trod the familiar route to PICU, gathering courage, aware of the pivotal hour to come. Heather would depart the hospital for the first time in her sixteen months. I felt no euphoria. I'd tucked her in each evening for fifty bedtimes, not so long really. Perhaps Jim and I would never see her again. We weren't yet licensed as foster parents.

The new foster mother scrubbed her hands and put on a cover gown. I introduced myself to Sue Wilson and gave a brief explanation. Her pregnancy created an easy opening for chit-chat. It was her impression that Heather would live with them for one or two months, then move to a state institution. She was happy to learn of our interest, better option than a state home.

With Heather, there would be five children in their home, the most HRS regulations allowed in a household. After Sue's baby was born, there'd be too many. Heather would have to go, but with an ongoing shortage of foster homes, HRS routinely overlooked their own guidelines.

"The state's providing round-the-clock in our home nurses for the first few days, and then continues it at sixteen hours a day. No need for special wiring or a generator," she said. She answered more of my questions. In theory Medicaid would cover all Heather's medical expenses until age eighteen, even if she was released from foster care through a permanent adoption.

"Come visit Heather. I've asked the PICU nurses to keep in touch too," Sue invited, scribbling down her phone number and handing it to me.

Later, Jim stopped by PICU to bid his farewell. He crossed paths with Sally, the nurse-specialist. "What are you doing here?" she asked, surprised.

"Saying 'bye,' we weren't licensed in time," Jim answered. "HRS didn't receive a rush request, so they didn't expedite the process."

"What a shame, but there are more babies like Heather. I thought you hadn't followed through," Sally said in a hushed voice.

Jim did not reply as her remark offered no comfort.

The next day Heather left the hospital with the Wilsons. They rolled her out in an over-sized wheelchair with padded braces and cushions to support her floppy body and head. Sparse hair lay soft on her head. Her expression and blush-colored lips unmoving in a perpetual pout.

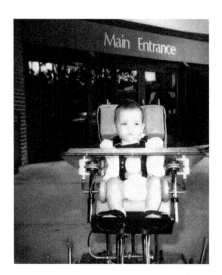

I waited a respectable week and acted on the foster-mother's invitation. Pulling into their driveway, a ponytailed girl shooting hoops hollered at her mom. Greeting her, I offered a baked casserole. "My grandmother's recipe—noodles and ground beef, tossed with mushroom and tomato soups, peppers, and onions. All topped with grated cheese. Delicious."

"A lot of nurses promised to call, but no others have," Sue Wilson said, stubbing out her cigarette. Inside in the living room, her four children skipped about. Heather rested in an infant seat, seemingly oblivious to the giggly, rambunctious commotion. "Having strangers here has my kids acting wild. Small Kurt hit Heather above her eyebrows, and a knot popped out," she said, pointing to the owie. "Poor thing can't even sound the quietest cry. Want to hold her?" she offered.

I hoisted frail Heather onto my hip, cupping my hand behind her head in case it wobbled. The blue dress accentuated the murky color of her skin. Perhaps it is better to dress her in pink, I thought. Heather didn't blink her eyes in greeting, and neither did I. Had she forgotten me? Was she angry?

Sue went on about her experiences. We sat down on a faded couch in her living room. I cherished holding Heather.

"Friday I almost sent her back to the hospital. Her care is too exhausting," Sue said. "The first nurses were experienced in caring for a child with a tracheotomy and gastrostomy tube, but the last RNs had never even seen a tracheotomy, much less cared for such a patient! They sleep or watch TV. They forget to turn on the alarms that monitor her heart and breathing." To emphasize her exasperation, she drummed the table top with her index finger. "At midnight I get off work, and then stay up all hours doing their job."

Framed pictures hung on the walls of the many foster children who had shared their home. "If one of these kids dies on me, I'll quit this," she groaned. "One baby came to us wrapped in foam, almost every bone broken. He lived here almost three years. We asked to adopt him, but HRS sent him back home to the perpetrator." She hesitated to collect her composure. "A high-school diploma is the only requirement for being a caseworker. Each child in a caseload is supposed to be checked on monthly, but in reality maybe happens once a year. Not enough staff."

"Can I help with something before I go?" I offered, not wanting to overstay my welcome.

"I'd be very grateful if you'd tidy this room. Please come again next week, and bring your daughter," she urged. I settled Heather into the infant seat and proceeded to put away a mess of scattered toys.

"Look how Heather watches you!" Sue exclaimed. "Her eyes follow you everywhere. It is obvious how much she loves you." We bid our good-byes.

Meanwhile, back at home, Jim concocted a surprise. That year was our tenth wedding anniversary.

A red hibiscus floated in a wide-necked crystal vase on a side table near the fireplace. Lettered in large print on a sheet of paper next to a cassette radio were the words, "PLAY ME. HAPPY ANNIVERSARY!" Charmed and intrigued, I listened to the message:

> "This recording will self-destruct. Your mission, should you choose to accept it, will transpire on November 11. At 6:00 p.m. a 'known stranger' will knock at your door. From that point, you will be addressed as the lovely Lady Ketterling. The reconnoiterer will transport you to an undisclosed destination. Attire is semiformal. One day prior to the mission, please report to your childhood home."

The background music was the theme song for "Mission Impossible"; the voice was my husband's. Baffled, I replayed it. Maybe one of those "Clue" parties, the whodunit game was a favorite, as were Agatha Christie mystery novels.

Jim acted ignorant.

"I don't like surprises," I said. "Kindly tell me what's up."

"Not a chance," he replied.

"A hint, pretty please." I smiled extra sweetly.

"You agree to the mission or not?" he quizzed.

"Of course, who wouldn't?"

"Better get used to mysteries," he teased, his eyes mischievous.

"Kids," I yelled. "Your dad is something else." We all laughed.

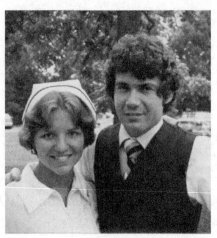

Ann's nursing school graduation, Florida State University
Engaged to James Gregory Giganti

Clandestine day arrived. As instructed, we'd driven to my parents' home. "What do your children like to eat for breakfast?" Mom asked, before leaving for the grocery store. She always aimed to please.

"Aren't I coming home?" I asked.

"Whoops!" she replied.

Midafternoon, Jim and the children bustled off to who knows where, leaving me several hours to leisurely dress.

Out back, my mom's garden path meandered past a frangipani cluster. I moseyed up the stairs of a rustic bamboo teahouse to its open rooftop deck. A great blue heron stalked fish in the river's edge. Schools of mullet bobbled over a shallow sandbar. Mangrove islands shielded us from the main Banana River.

I daydreamed; maybe Jim and I would embark on a cruise out of the port. Back inside, I showered, put on a robe, and began ironing a colorful cocktail dress. Unpinning the hot rollers in my hair one by one, I stood under the air-conditioning vent to cool the waves.

The doorbell chimed. I didn't answer as Jim could use his key. I pulled on a slip and then my dress. The bell rang again. I ran to the door and peeked out the window. It wasn't Jim. It was a tall lady wearing an elegant plumed hat, large sunglasses, and a trench coat with the collar turned up so it concealed her neck.

"Kristin!" I greeted my sister.

"*Bon jour*, Lady Ketterling," she said. "Let me introduce myself; my name is Madame Merganser." She gestured toward a new-model car. Hers, not ours.

"Kristin, I am not ready," I said.

"You have mistaken my identity. I am Madame Merganser. I recently arrived from the West Indies," she said with a faint French accent.

"One moment, I'll be right back." I fastened my hair with a jeweled barrette and let curls fall to my shoulders. I slid into sheer stockings and coral satin pumps.

My chauffeur headed south on State Road A1A. Madame pulled into a grass-covered parking lot. In silence I followed her long strides down the sidewalk. Bright royal blue awnings shaded store windows, the restaurant's façade was a paneling of knotty driftwood.

What an odd pair, Madame in her mysterious getup and me dressed as spring flowers. She tugged open a heavy wooden door and ushered me into Bernard's Surf. "Reservations for Lady Ketterling," she said to the doorman, then tipped her feathered hat and departed.

"The gentleman is waiting," the hostess said and escorted me to the nautical room. At a candlelit table sat my clever husband. Ten years earlier, Jim's father, Geno, had hosted our rehearsal dinner in the exact same room, bestowing wishes for a long and joyful marriage.

"You are the best! Perhaps I could learn to like surprises." I thanked my husband. We didn't want the weekend to end, but of course, it did.

A week later I went to the Wilsons. Jamie came with me and was so excited to finally meet Heather. Fear attacked when we entered their home. The polluted atmosphere triggered a cramping uneasiness. During the night outdoor temperature dropped to below freezing. Heated air blasted from the heating vents, and all windows were tightly closed. Smoke clouded the living room. A burning cigarette dangled from Sue's hand, same issue, more lit smokes in the hands of her two friends.

"I hide the ashtrays when any caseworker comes," Sue remarked in an offhanded way. We exchanged superficial greetings. She must not have noticed my initial furtive glances.

Would Heather's damaged lungs be able to cope with the added threat? Should I speak up or keep mum? Our attorney had clearly explained that we'd need the Wilsons' blessings if we were to eventually adopt Heather.

"I'm exhausted. Heather needs breathing treatments every two hours and tube feedings every four. She's due now. For a favor would you administer both?"

"Sure," I answered.

After providing the therapies, Jamie and I took Heather outside to the side yard. In the sunshine the temp climbed back into the 70s. Sitting down atop a picnic table, a cardinal flitting the lower limbs of a sycamore tree scolded us for coming too close.

Heather wouldn't respond to my eye blinks.

Jamie snugged her close. A tiny yellowish bug with glistening spots of black lighted on Heather's wrist. It flicked open and closed its outer hard-shell wings. "Keep still, let's watch the pretty insect," Jamie coaxed. Becoming aware of the uninvited visitor, Heather fidgeted, and the bug flew off.

The rumble and clatter of an old truck disturbed the quiet, followed by a whir of larger machinery. Jamie carried Heather to the fence to more closely observe the action in the yard

across the street. They gazed at the weed-eater, spinning up foot-high whirls of grass and dirt. An older man revved up an edger. Its blades struck the driveway; sparks showered like spraying fireworks. A third fellow rode in comfort on a wide-seated lawn mower.

A breeze picked up and tousled Jamie's thick ringlets and Heather's fine hair. "She's so sweet," Jamie said, "I hope she gets to be my sister."

Apprehension about the cigarettes continued its torment during the hour's drive home. I turned to Celeste for advice; talking with her always generated renewed strength.

"If she's pregnant and hasn't quit smoking, she'll not worry about Heather," Celeste said.

It seemed the only option was to speak with the nurse-specialist. "Sally," I said, "there's a problem. . . ."

"The Wilsons assured us that they'd smoke outside." Sally sounded distraught. "All I can do is to remind her. Don't worry, I'll be subtle and won't mention any names," she promised. "By the way, Sue says Heather responds really well to you. And relax, there's no institution that will take her; or she'd have been sent there long ago."

CHAPTER 9] WAKE-UP NUDGE

Six days later I drove to the Wilsons. Long lines of crows rested on the power lines strung along the country road. A little farther along, skittish buzzards obstructed my passage and hopped about in staccato leaps. They acted reluctant to leave a road kill; not feeding on the dead animal, just hovering around it, rising in abrupt flights and landing only a foot or two away. I slowed to avoid striking any of them. Behind me the horns of an eighteen-wheeler and a single car blared. Steering to the left of the bird mob, I discovered the seeming reason for the odd behavior. It was one of their own that had been struck, in death resembling a collapsed sack of silken black feathers.

I pulled into Sue's driveway and waved.

"You'll spoil me," she said, accepting my offering of various casseroles. She beckoned me to follow her into the kitchen and placed the tasty dishes on the counter top.

From under folded newspapers she withdrew a book of matches, opening and shutting the packet several times before striking a light and touching the flame to her cigarette. She inhaled a long drag, exhaling a cloud. Nonplussed, I detoured my staring scrutiny to a random blemish on the ceiling. I guess I failed because Sue stubbed out the cigarette and fanned the smoke.

"Suzy tried dabbing a drop of chocolate pudding onto Heather's tongue, but nothing happened, no moving of her lips or swallowing. She managed to teach Heather to sit. Sometimes she topples."

"That's wonderful progress," I complimented, focusing on the genuine accomplishment.

Sue's next comment seemed miraculous. "After Christmas Heather can move to your home; best do it before I get too attached. Call my supervisor, Cindy Smith, and find out how we go about it."

Early the next morning, Sue called me, talking frantic. "They've scaled back the in-home nurses' hours. I can't keep the pace, with my morning sickness. Have you talked to Cindy? If Heather goes to you, my husband and I can provide shelter for a less complicated child."

"Cindy's office is closed," I answered.

"Please call as soon as they open, and contact Children's Medical Services (CMS)," she begged. "Have you received your official foster-parent license in the mail yet?" she asked. No paper license, but we were formally approved. I was confused as to why if we were approved, the paper stamped license was so critical, but it seemed much hedged on it.

Once I had more information, Sue and I conferred. CMS recommended moving Heather to our home after her next monthly bronchoscopy. Tiny buds of glory sprouted as Jim and I anticipated a joyful homecoming.

Hiring a medically skilled babysitter would likely be impossible. To lessen the financial impact, Jim and I planned to work opposite shifts so one of us would always be available to care for Heather. My supervisor agreed to schedule me to work the short four-hour evening shifts or Saturday and Sunday twelve-hour days.

In the highest of spirits, Jim drove us to Whitley's Christmas Tree Farm on a hunt for the perfect red cedar from evergreens. A cool breeze stirred their needles in a soft rustling melody. The owner's weathered face crinkled merrily as he observed Jamie and Tony racing zigzag about his trails. At last they selected a plump one with widely spaced branches. Were we dreaming, or might Heather soon join in our Yuletide dreams?

All too soon snipped by a disquieting call from Cindy Smith. "Now don't get upset," she implored. "It'll work out. No more visiting Heather at the Wilsons' home. Too much negative gossip about the foster family." She didn't provide specifics on who was gossiping. "Lie low, then no one can blame you."

Shaken. Devastated. Maybe I'd misread Sue. Yet Sue insisted that the no-visit order hadn't come from her. Bewildered, Jim and I speculated about what might have gone wrong. The specialist promised to be discreet about the cigarette issue and truly loved Heather.

Moving forward, Jim and I would only trust long-term friends who were in no way associated with the hospital or HRS.

We called our attorney for guidance.

"When is the next bronchoscopy?" Martha asked.

"It's coming up soon," I answered.

"Did anyone say you couldn't go?" she asked.

"No one told us not to go to the hospital," I said.

"You can catch up with Heather there," she recommended. "In the meantime, compile an album with lots of family and neighborhood photos. Drive the few hours to the Park County HRS office and plan on spending the whole day. Don't call for an appointment ahead, as Cindy Smith might refuse point blank. If she isn't there, just leave.

Without making yourself a nuisance, keep returning until you can introduce yourself and hand her the photo album. The goal is becoming an actual person to her, not just a voice on the phone. Luck may have Cindy invite you to stay and chat for a while."

On the day of the trek, Celeste babysat Tony. If I had to fritter away the entire day, hanging out near the Park County HRS … trying not to be a pest, Jamie would get dropped there after school.

I arrived mid-morning and jotted down her office number in case it floated out of my nervous mind. A plump middle-aged woman strode purposefully down the hall. Timorous about my soon-to-be meeting with Heather's assigned social worker, I caught her gaze and smiled despite preferring to stare at the floor. The door to room 112 was ajar. No one was in there.

I hurried toward the sound of a file drawer squeaking open, then hesitated until I could muster a cheerful facade.

"Excuse me," I said to a tall man wearing a collared shirt and plain necktie. "I'm looking for Cindy Smith."

"She'll be right back. You can wait in her office," he suggested. "There's a comfortable chair next to the window." I felt giddy with anticipation. Maybe, just maybe, Cindy Smith would be the key to bringing Heather home.

Books stood haphazardly on built-in shelving that lined the walls. Purple wildflowers spilled from a pottery vase on the desk. I took a peppermint from a crystal candy bowl. I flipped through the album I'd compiled to portray our family. There were photographs of Jim and me and the kids acting silly on a porch swing, Mom churning ice cream on Jamie's eighth birthday, cousins wading the cold-water stream at Groundhog Flats, and one of my frail grandfather playing the piano with gusto to entertain my young children. I'd snapped photos of each room in our home, including the two bathrooms, and provided copies of our employment evaluations and Jamie's school report cards.

What a surprise when the woman who had smiled at me in the hallway walked in and sat down behind the desk. She was Cindy Smith, the social worker whom I had come to meet. "We've talked about Heather," I said and handed her the album and a small burlap sack of unshelled pecans.

"You brought these for me?" Her sturdy face went soft and friendly, and her attention shifted to the album.

"Hand-written notes explain each picture," I said. "Your schedule's busy." I stood to leave.

"Stay a few minutes," she invited and began thumbing through the pages while I related favorite family stories. "Follow me please," she directed. As we entered the adoption supervisor's office, the clicking of typewriter keys ceased. Diane Morris looked up at us, resting her elbows on the desk. After listening for a few moments, she eased back in her swivel chair and swung around, clapping her hands in delight.

"I remember you! Your timing is fortunate," she exclaimed. "Her case came across my desk. Now we can avoid searching the whole state for adoptive parents. It would be appropriate to move Heather to you as a foster child until you and your husband can complete the HRS series of adoption classes. Undergoing a new family investigation won't be necessary."

She closed the album and started to hand it back.

"Perhaps keep it for your records?" I suggested.

Ecstatic at such positive feedback, the drive home seemed only minutes. I shared my enthusiasm with Jim's parents, who were visiting for a week. "I'm from the old school. I say it how I see it," Geno said. "If she remains handicapped, she'll cause great financial hardship." His adamant doubts couldn't squelch our enthusiasm.

The radio played Burl Ives's "The Twelve Days of Christmas." Spiced apple cider mulled on the stove. My brother Mike came over for holiday cookie making. He layered fat lighter, dry twigs, and oak logs in the fireplace, and a blaze soon crackled.

In the kitchen, we mashed together a jumbo jar of peanut butter, a pound of margarine, and two pounds of powdered sugar. Sticky fingers hand-rolled gooey globs of sweetness into balls and dipped them into melted chocolate.

Putting on festive attire, we began going door-to-door, handing out the deliciousness to neighbors. Half the fun was walking under the glorious night sky. Stopping at the Hoffenbergs, we insisted that Mark, Celeste, and Haley come along. "Please, please. We've seen seven shooting stars."

"Bring a sweater," I suggested, and then shared a disappointment with Celeste. Intermixed with holiday greeting cards, I'd spotted a letter from HRS. Into my lap fell the vital paper foster-parent license, embossed with Florida's Official Seal. "The 'official license' is no trump card," I said. Thinking it would expedite moving Heather to our home, I'd spoken to all appropriate people, but no one had called me back with a definitive plan. Too much bureaucracy, I figured.

"The system's operating under 'don't rock the boat,' because instead of getting a smoother ride, the boat might sink. No guarantees that something pretty might be a fake. I know you and Jim, HRS doesn't," Celeste commiserated.

"Status quo, no one of power is pushing for the move. A baby can't complain," I said.

"The Masons are an improvement from the hospital." Jim said, inserting a rational perspective. "Ann and I are the main people wanting to speed up the move. It's best if we become her permanent parents. We'll suffer the consequences of any miscalculations in her care."

The quest didn't get easier. I took to pretending to be patient; I took to more strumming of the guitar and silent prayers. Maybe, just maybe, one day.

Heather returned to PICU for another of those monthly bronchoscopic examinations and tracheal dilations. Jim followed our attorney's advice and went there to visit Heather. Something went sour. Entering our house, he oozed palpable tension. That little muscle near his right ear twitched. I'd never seen him so peculiarly out-of-sorts.

"When I showed my visitor's pass," he said, "the PICU clerk fidgeted, then paged the charge nurse. That lady stalled, performing a few tasks, then spoke about trivia, evading the real message. She finally stammered out the directives in a polite way—HRS was prohibiting any visitors to Heather. The only exception is the current foster family."

"Better you turned away than me," I said. "My composure might have disappeared into a melt-down quicker than a thwarted two-year-old can throw a tantrum." Baffled at the turn of events, defeat rushed in, getting a grip.

In a search for a logical explanation, Jim had me telephone a PICU nurse who was an acquaintance of ours. She refused to give specific details. "Don't trust anybody," she warned. "At each shift change an administrator apprises the staff that it's illegal to divulge any information. They cite your names specifically, twisting it as if you and Jim are some kind of crazies."

Devastated, Jim and I were knocked down to the essence: keeping faith in an unseen and mysterious guidance that somehow kept us plodding along. I collapsed on the couch, curled up on my side, and covered myself with a cozy afghan, wanting to drift into a deep sleep and fantasy world of happy dreams.

Christmas morning my mother-in-law popped the cork off a champagne bottle and toasted the beginning of festivities. Cinnamon buns baked in the oven. After a fast-paced opening of holiday gifts, five bow-tied packages conspicuously remained (for Heather and Sue's children). Each a reminder of the absence of our hoped-for new daughter. We enjoyed the comfort and commotion of our family traditions.

New Years came and went. There was still no news of Heather. On January 23, desperate for a nap, I'd refreshed my bed with newly washed sheets and snuggled under the blankets. Tony was already snoozing, and Jamie was studying spelling words. "Please don't disturb me, I'm exhausted. Take a message if anyone calls," I directed. Not sure how much time had passed, when Jamie's little hand gently rubbed my shoulder to rouse me.

"Mom," Jamie whispered. "The lady on the phone says to wake you; it is very important." She handed me the receiver.

"Hello." My voice creaked with sleep.

"Do you still want Heather?" a hesitant voice asked.

"Absolutely," I eased off the bed and shook my arms and legs and stretched a little to hasten wakefulness.

"The Wilsons are frayed and want her out." The harried social worker spelled out the situation. "Heather's been admitted to the hospital. Can you and Jim go there first thing tomorrow to begin medical training?"

"Of course. Is she okay?"

"Just another bronchoscopy. Her nurse will call with instructions. Thanks," she said.

Jim and I wondered how whoever-had-previously-blocked-our-visits would react to the turn of events.

CHAPTER 10] STAYING ALIVE

Relief almost sent me backflipping across the moon. "Heather is coming home!" I sang the joyous words. With jolliness, Jamie, Tony, and I danced around, cranking up some reggae songs. Jim arranged taking time off from his work for the medical training sessions. Trachs are risky business. Neck-breathing bypasses many protective reflexes. Water can fill the lungs unchecked, resulting in drowning. Outdoors, crawly bugs and blowing sand are a persistent threat. The gag reflex is bypassed, icky things can be inhaled leading to abscess and infection in the lungs.

A pulmonary nurse clinician would be our go-to person. Letters went out to the fire department and electric company to apprise them of Heather's medical condition and gave our home priority status in case of a wide-spread power outage.

Promptly at 9:00 a.m., Jim and I strode the familiar hospital path, scrubbed our hands with germicidal soap, donned our gowns, and settled in to enjoy the nearness of sweet sleeping Heather. A sour-faced nurse trudged our way. "Policy forbids any morning visitors," she scolded and gestured for us to leave.

"Bob specifically instructed that we wait by Heather's crib," Jim explained about the teaching session in his peace-making voice. No additional words were necessary. Good fortune arrived in the shape of a large, bearded nurse. His arms were loaded with supplies. Bob was tasked with instructing us in all the nuances and lethality of tracheotomy care and related medical procedures.

"An emergency delayed me." He uttered an apology, then briefed us on his professional qualifications and spoke a little about his family. We reciprocated, following the unwritten protocol of establishing credentials and exchanging pleasantries.

Trachs are life-saving and lethal. For Heather, since making sound with her vocal cords was impossible, total occlusion with mucous caused inaudible asphyxiation that progressed until oxygen deprivation slowed her heart beats enough to trigger a bradycardia (slow heart beat) alarm. When that happened, lifesaving measures had to begin within seconds.

Heather's neck-breathing bypassed her nose and went in dry directly to the lungs. For most people the nose humidifies, warms, and filters inhaled breaths. Breathing dry air evaporated moisture from the thin mucous puddling in her trach tube, drying it into hard plugs. Whistling breaths warned of such impending obstructive catastrophes and required an emergency trach change.

Dusty unfiltered air often irritated the tiny alveoli air sacs. Her lungs produced copious secretions in an attempt at cleansing themselves. To assist her, while in the crib or at night, the air she breathed was moistened by a compressor bubbling it through sterile water. Corrugated plastic tubing channeled the cool mist so it would blow into a mask placed loosely over Heather's trach, so she could inhale it.

Jim asked Bob about the actual feel of a trach change, the removal of the old one and insertion of a clean one. "Some kids think it's like bad brute Joe punched them in the chest. Others aren't affected."

Bob captured our total attention, and we listened to his warnings as if he were Moses. Anything can happen. "Once when we tugged the dirty trach tube out of a teenager's neck, she bolted, then raced berserk around until collapsing. Her windpipe had spasmed so tightly that a clean trach tube could not be slipped back in, not even the smallest one. She died."

Foam ties that fasten with Velcro are to be avoided because curious child fingers can grasp at the pointy corners and tug them loose. Unfastened trach ties create a trach-falls-out disaster. Preferred are twill cloth ties to snug a trach in place. Using a baby doll model, Bob located the holes in the trach's side flanges, pulled the ties through, wrapped them snugly around the doll's neck, and knotted securely.

"It takes two people to safely change a trach. Once when everybody was too busy, I forged ahead solo. Nothing to it, piece of cake," Bob pantomimed cockiness. "I snipped the ties, pulled out the old trach, and pushed in a clean one. The little guy coughed, the not-yet-tied-in-place trach tube jettisoned onto the floor. Big problem, I reached for the spare clean tube that is kept taped to the bed. It wasn't there! Gagging, I plucked the wayward dirty tube off the floor and plunged it back into the toddler's neck. Nasty, but he couldn't breathe without it."

In the morning, there would be more sessions. As we left for the day, a respiratory therapist handed over a staggering list of essential supplies.

Exhausted and exhilarated, and as a time-saver, we splurged and ordered pizza. Organizing space for Heather's medical equipment and supplies assumed top priority. Jim raised the mattress in the crib to its highest position. It was the same one Jamie and Tony had slept in as babies.

After a while I took a break from preparations and returned to the PICU to read Heather bedtime stories. I gathered her up, hearing and feeling the slight gurgle that often accompanied each of her breaths.

"You want two?" The question of a pretty young nurse startled me.

I shrugged my shoulders, not comprehending.

"Alexander's foster parents returned him," she confided. "Caring for him and his trach exhausted them and stressed their marriage to the verge of divorce." Sturdy Alexander toddled over. "You remember Heather," the pretty nurse said and tousled his hair.

"One's enough," I squeaked. How could his foster parents dump him? If two experienced PICU nurses couldn't muster the energy to be mom, dad, and nurse to Alexander, a boy who had a trach, but could run and eat then how could Jim and I possibly succeed? Inexperienced as parents, I rationalized. They'd underestimated the work in parenting two toddlers, doubly so if one has special needs.

"Maybe, would you give Heather her bath?" the same pretty nurse suggested. She ran an inch of tepid water in the sink. "No deeper or water will seep through the feeding hole into her belly. Be especially careful of the trach."

From her big toe I tenderly untaped the glowing red light sensor that measured the oxygen content in her blood. Off came her soiled shirt. Dried trach spittle stiffened its front. I peeled off three sticky chest patches that attached to wires monitoring her heart and breathing rates. To keep her intravenous site dry, I covered it with a plastic bag.

Undressed, her head looked too big for her spindly body. I wrung out a soapy washcloth and sponged clean her neck and skinny arms, legs, and rounded belly. With a fluffy towel, I dried her.

After clothing her, I settled her into a walker. She no longer needed propping with the teddy bear. Quick as a crab, she scurried sideways, silent happiness spilling everywhere. A twill-tape tether leashed the walker to the crib lest she escape down the hall. I sat down on the floor, and she scooted over to me, eyes blinking happily.

After two days of instruction, testing time came to determine how Jim and I might handle emergencies. "Okay if I get a drink of water?" I asked Bob.

"Nervous cotton-mouth," he teased.

I'd been a nurse for more than ten years, but it was harder to concentrate with Heather's future at stake. Expertly Jim and I each demonstrated cardiopulmonary resuscitation on the model baby doll. Next station was alive and feeling Heather and a real trach change in her precious living airway, not practicing on a plastic mannequin.

Jim laid her on a baby blanket. He grasped the upper left corner, drew it over her left shoulder and arm and tucked it under her back, pinning the arm to her side. He did the same with her right arm. I took a longer blanket, folded it in half lengthwise, and wrapped it around her torso and legs so she looked like a cocoon with a head poking out. A small washcloth roll tucked under her neck tilted back her head for an easier view of the neck and trach.

Jim toggled on the suction machine, and it rattled to life. He checked connections for leaks and pinched off the tubing to adjust its maximum pressure to 100 mm Hg. He laid out three catheters, confirmed location of the spare trachs (same size and one smaller), and connected oxygen tubing to a manual ventilation bag in case Heather needed hand-squeezed breaths.

I cut two six-inch cloth ties to diagonal points. My fingers felt as stubby and awkward as toes when I tried to push each tip through the tiny flange openings to secure them to the new trach. We scrubbed our hands once more, and Jim donned sterile gloves. Heather's papoosed body waited quietly, and she looked at us with calm, patient trust.

Jim suctioned excess secretions from inside her old trach so they wouldn't puddle and obscure our landmarks. The idea of invading her body disturbed him. Beads of sweat dripped off his forehead. He knew minutes of delay in reinserting a trach could cause asphyxiation, brain damage, and death. His juxtaposed fingers held the in-place trach gently but firmly against Heather's neck while I snipped the ties. That done, I grasped the new trach in my right hand.

"Good thing this is a low-stress situation," my husband joked. "Ready?"

My body felt like melting jelly, but I nodded.

Jim removed the tube, and the neck hole closed. With a swift arcing motion I placed the new one with trailing attached ties into the dimple that remained and held it snug to her neck while Jim lifted her head, wrapped the ties around her neck and tied a knot. We would leave them long as a visual reminder recheck for any stretching.

After an hour passed, we'd retie them more snugly if needed, then cut off the excess. Heather hadn't reacted to any of the intrusive procedures. After freeing her from the blankets, I hugged her tight. Jim and I felt drained and at the same time euphoric, as if having just run a marathon. Bob applauded our success.

After her bronchoscopy the next morning, and a following full day of recovery, Heather would at last come home. Was it a dreamy charade or solid fact?

Envisioning a happy and hectic week, we brought home two cartloads of groceries. Celeste selected a date for a baby shower and went shopping for decorations. My parents packed their suitcases in eager anticipation of arriving to embrace their new granddaughter on the first weekend of her homecoming.

Three hours later via the telephone, unpleasant words felled us like the quick strike of a cobra. "You can't have her," the social worker said. She didn't elaborate. The bad news crushed Jamie and Tony, silenced Jim, and tossed me into a bleak abyss.

Heather again left the hospital with the Wilsons. Doubt that she'd ever join our family submerged us in a gloom deeper than the unexplored ocean floor. Senseless adoption games and their vexing players had finally worn us down. Bewildered, we turned to the Catholic Church. Weekend work had been partial reasoning for sporadic attendance. Our spiritual beliefs gave us enough strength. We'd thought that weekly organized religion was for other people.

Nevertheless, on the Sunday following Heather's thwarted homecoming, Jim and I dressed the children in their best and headed for church. On our knees we asked God for guidance and the strength to persist. A call received a week later whittled us down to subsisting on the essence of a faith deep in our core, passed down from generations of church-goers.

"Heather's hospitalized," relayed the somber social worker. "If she recovers, she'll go home with your family."

"Can we go to her, right now?" I asked.

"The faster the better."

"What happened?"

"Ask the doctor," she responded in a too soft voice. Panic set in. Was Heather dying?

The sight of Heather seared us like a molten rod. Her skin was a ghostly gray even with high levels of supplemental oxygen. Infection racked her scarred lungs. She focused murky, drifting eyes on Jim while taking torturous breaths. She didn't seem to respond to our words or gentle touch. What did she remember? We wondered if she had missed us or thought the hospital was again her eternal home.

"Heather might always require supplemental oxygen," the doctor warned. Unwilling to grapple with the notion of forever chaining her to an oxygen tank, we discounted the possibility, instead framing her situation as an acute setback. Six days slid by with Heather teetering near death. To ward off despair we reflected on her exuberant scooting in her baby walker that we'd observed during our training and daydreamed of the day she would clutch a toy in her fingers, break into a smile, and share a loving hug.

"What's going on? There are a lot of rumors." Sue Wilson called me, distraught.

"HRS said you wanted Heather moved to our home," I answered.

"My husband requested better qualified in-home nurses, that is all," she corrected. "Keep us posted, will you?"

Thankfully Heather improved and weaned off the oxygen. They promised no more glitches. I updated our attorney. The whole neighborhood effervesced with joy. A flurry of activity ensued. Supply companies piled a mountain of medical stuff in our living room. Were we nuts? Jim and I made our way to the hospital, minds awhirl with terror that some unknown might again pull the rug out from under the dream.

CHAPTER 11] JOYFUL PROGRESS

Thursday, February 16, 1989, Heather came home as our foster daughter. Without continuous surveillance, Heather would die. Would Jim and I be savvy and lucky enough to keep her alive?

PICU celebrated like a jolly carnival. Happy nurses crowded around. An older one snapped pictures. I slipped ethereal, eighteen-month-old Heather into a one-year-size dress that dwarfed her twelve-pound frame. Yes, the rosy color brought out the pink tones in her complexion.

A medical bag would shadow Heather everywhere. Jim packed it with an emergency trach-change kit, resuscitative supplies, heart and breathing alarms, and battery-operated suction and nebulizing machines. Bob once more drilled key instructions. "Asphyxiation is the biggest danger. Keep the trach tube clear of mucous as she's too weak to cough out thin or thick secretions. Remember if the tube gets plugged or falls out, she'll die in fewer than five minutes."

All wished us luck as we waved good-bye and pushed Heather in a stroller out of PICU and into the corridor. Temporary or permanent parents, we'd discover our fate as it unfolded. An abundance of joy or learning to find peace in heartache, that too remained to be determined. Proud Jim sauntered along. We detoured and stopped by his office to show off our frail daughter.

Such an overload of commotion, yet Heather's base response was the quiet repose of a newborn.

Our old blue Mercury carried us home; and though it wasn't a magical pumpkin turned fanciful carriage, I felt like Heather's fairy godmother and hoped that Jim and I might cast an enchanted spell transforming her life. The surroundings were not as ornate as Cinderella's castle, but our aspirations were loftier than royalty and riches.

Newly a big brother, Tony burst out the front door pulling a wagonload of toys. I balanced Heather on my knee for their pivotal meeting. Her heartbeat quickened under the lace. She straightened her droopy head, riveting attention on her sibling as he chattered nonstop.

I shuddered to think her being there might be a mirage and trembled because it was not. No longer fearing her placement in an institution, Jim and I contemplated what we had done—taken in a very sick little girl, and perhaps, maybe we were indeed crazy.

That afternoon was a grand open house of people and emotions. Respiratory therapists, medical suppliers, supervisory nurses, and friends paraded through our home. Immediate explanations of Heather's condition prevented the awkwardness of unspoken questions.

Quiet Heather sat motionless in a baby seat except for the burdened rise and fall of her chest. She no longer required the assistance of a ventilator, but each breath was a struggle. The muscles in her neck strained, the skin pulled in between her ribs, and her abdomen pumped.

Neighborhood kids stared at the thin tube dripping nourishment. I showed them how it hooked into the feeding button in her belly and how it provided all her sustenance. With fervor I warned against messing with the button or trach. Bob had cautioned about curious playmates who might yank on a feeding-button as it resembled an air-mattress plug, thinking the child might deflate like a beach ball.

I contacted Sue once things settled down.

"Ann, HRS never notified us about the move. Good thing we stayed friends, despite the gossip. All her belongings are here." Sue sounded discouraged.

"She made amazing progress under your care," I said. Under their guidance, she'd learned to hold her head more erect, sit without propping, and manage a slow, feeble crawl. Attempts to teach her to drink fluid from a bottle or cup or to eat food by mouth had failed.

Heather wasn't a solitary package. The mandatory in-our-home night nurses were arranged by an agency the hospital selected. Day nurses were offered. We declined more invasion of our family life. Having a stranger overnight in the girls' room, directly across from ours, seemed awkward enough, but Jim and I did require some sleep.

After the Wilsons' stories, the whole idea generated apprehension. Would the nurses be skilled or deceptive? Might they turn off annoying but vital alarms? Some could purposefully or accidentally take the easy option and snooze the night away. Maybe in ignorance they'd suction too long depriving Heather of taking in breaths or withdrawing air from her lungs to the point of deflation. Deep suctioning can suck in airway tissue and tear it away with bleeding and scarring.

Driving the school carpool would be infinitely easier if I could leave Heather and all her equipment at home. We asked the night nurses to stay until I returned. Some awake time with Heather might prevent wrong conclusions and their mislabeling her "vegetable."

Doorbell chimes announced the arrival of the first night nurse, middle-aged Laura. Already in pajamas, shyly Jamie and Tony scooted around and crouched down behind and alongside the arm of the oversized chair and peered up at her standing in the doorway.

"I'm afraid you're early, can we trouble you to return at 11 p.m.?" Jim asked.

"The agency told me to arrive at 8:00 p.m.," she insisted.

"Sorry for any miscommunication. Please understand, the later hour prevents interruptions to the bedtime routine." He started shutting the door.

"Before I leave, can I tell Heather a quick 'hello'?" she asked. Laura greeted the whimsical child with affection. "Might not need me so much, you have a family now," she said.

Jamie and Heather's room bore the countenance of both a pediatric intensive-care unit and a girl's room. Jamie voiced her dissent. "It'll be weird to sleep with a stranger sitting near me. Can't I sleep in the extra bed in Tony's room?"

"You are so right; that's a terrific idea. Time for bed," Jim said.

When Laura returned, I escorted her to Heather already asleep in the crib, and reviewed her care in detail. I mentioned and pointed out the large sign taped on the crib: "Trach-tie changes to be performed by parents only." Jim and I elected to do that task ourselves, as we had more at stake than the nurses on duty. I showed her the location of equipment and supplies and gave a quick house tour, including the important refrigerator and bathroom. I invited her to please feel welcome and comfortable.

With multiple caregivers, I tried to make it simple. On the desk, a clipboard displayed a typed list of house rules for the on-duty nurse to read. Nearby was a spiral communication book where I'd write updates or new instructions. Anyone could jot down observations, ideas, or concerns.

New sounds filled the house—the noisy motor of the humidifying compressor, sporadic alarms, Heather's sputtering gurgles, and the whir of the suction machine. Too keyed up to sleep, I brewed a honey-ginger tea before crumpling into bed.

My parents arrived the next evening. Jim sprinted to greet them, expressing exuberance and relief. "Twenty-four hours has passed, and Heather's still alive!" We prayed for one more day of living, and then would pray for another, until a full week of survival; then keep on praying for additional weeks until voilà! A glorious first year.

Mom and Dad fell instantly in love with Heather. Until that moment they'd only heard descriptions, never seen any photos. "She appears healthier than I expected," Mom said, too kind to mention limp, spindly arms, bluish complexion, dark-circled eyes, or belly skin stretched tautly over an abdomen that bulged with insufficient room.

Dad contemplated that perhaps we weren't so crazy. His sister, Jo, had suffered with polio muscle paralysis as a young girl. Just in case her breathing muscles quit working, his Grandpa Kessler bought an iron-lung, one of only a few that existed in all of Kansas. Fortunately Aunt Jo never had to reside inside the whole person respirator that pumped your entire body to ventilate your lungs. Ravages of the disease shriveled her leg muscles.

The town's firemen devised an ingenious way for Jo to do water exercises to strengthen her legs. They hauled a horse's metal watering trough into the family's living room. Each day the dedicated men came with their truck and hoses to drain the trough's water and pump in fresh. Aunt Jo recovered except that one of her legs is shorter and weaker.

Dad asked when Heather might talk; never, unless, maybe someday, air could exit through her vocal cords. Then and only then, she had a chance of talking. If necessary, with the aid of a speaking valve, if sick lungs or muscle weakness made her forever inhale through the trach. Neck breathing is three times easier than breathing through the nose.

Perhaps Heather would never talk. If so, we would have to learn American Sign Language to communicate. The enormity of the task daunted us.

The second night brought a different kind of nurse knocking on our door. The stern individual was thin with hair drawn tightly into a bun, starched white dress and nursing cap, and spotless shoes. I spent an hour orienting her, same as I'd done with Laura.

Mom caught my attention and whispered, "She seems strange; nurses don't dress that way anymore. I couldn't get a conversation going with her; she wouldn't answer."

Looking in on Heather, there sat the reserved nurse with impeccable posture in a hard-back chair, reading a book perched on her lap. Heather slept in her crib, peaceful and cute in a pastel terry sleeper. I listened for the cadence of the usual soft gurgling sounds of her breathing. Properly functioning indicator lights of the heart and breathing monitors blinked reassuringly.

My parents, Jim, and I watched a televised comedy club show in the living room prior to our going to bed. Wonderful aromas of bacon, pancakes, and coffee teased us awake in the morning. "Come and get it," Dad called. After stuffing ourselves, we lounged around reading the Saturday comics. Heather was still sleeping in her crib.

From down the hallway, Jim's piercing cry struck like a lightning bolt heralding a tsunami. "The trach is out!" he shrieked. Already a horrid dusky blue color, Heather's chest muscles worked like bellows but couldn't inhale any air through the collapsed hole in her neck. Jim scanned the carpet, plucked up the plastic trach tube and placed it back into Heather's neck, opening her airway. His fingers held the wayward trach in place. Her frantic breaths could then draw in sweet, blessed air, and her skin pinked up.

"Mom, please get the emergency kit! It's on the dresser." She retrieved it and removed the lid.

Mom's fingers now held the wayward trach in Heather's neck. Jim used scissors from the kit to cut Heather's sleeper down the front to bare her chest and neck to make all landmarks more easily visible. Jim and I papoose-wrapped her with a small sheet from the kit. We deftly switched out the dirty trach with a clean one, and Jim meticulously knotted the ties. He left them long as we had been taught. In an hour we rechecked the twill ties, snugged the stretch out, retied and trimmed the excess. Jim's gentle expertise won my complete confidence.

Despite the spoken and posted prohibition, the strange nurse had changed the soiled trach ties, and had done so improperly. One flange was missing a tie, and the other was knotted ineffectively. The strange nurse acted unaware of the commotion. "Do you have any clean crib sheets?" she inquired.

"Heather's trach fell out." I said, scrubbing at tears flowing down my cheeks. "Your knots came undone. I told you not to change the trach ties. There is a sign posted on the bed. Worse is that you let her crawl around unobserved. She has no way to summon help."

"Where are the clean sheets?" she repeated, ignoring all I said. She finished charting, collected her purse, and left. I stiffened at her icy foul indifference that lingered even though she was gone. In her crisp uniform and cap and bizarre attitude, she reminded me of the Grim Reaper.

"Since she was neither comprehending, nor remorseful, she'll never again set foot in this house," I declared, and slumped into a chair.

"Going to be tough to love this granddaughter, so quickly might you lose her." My dad wept, voice and hands shaky. He realized there was no turning back, and the folly of his prior advice.

Reading the nurse's notes shattered us to the bone. It made it seem as though her scary actions had been deliberate, that she wished to cause Heather harm. Miss Coldheart had blatantly lied. She wrote that Jim and I had changed the ties and that she had assisted with replacing the wayward trach.

"Don't ever send that one back," Jim commanded when he reported the incident to the agency. Quivering in disbelief at the dreadful happening, we skedaddled out to the front yard for fresh air.

We soon learned it was not the strange nurse's only offense.

Celeste's sister introduced me to her co-worker whose young son had a trach. He too had narrowly escaped the "Grim Reaper nurse," who'd haunted their house with the same trick of failed trach knots. Invisible gates had opened, beckoning me to join a unique sisterhood, one that I never knew existed.

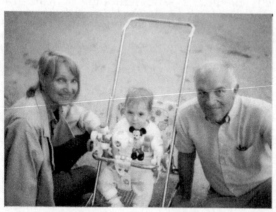

Heather with Ann's parents, Kathi and Fritz Widick

CHAPTER 12] ALL IN A DAY

Pleasant nurse Melissa came the third night. With vigor I detailed Heather's care, emphasizing the morning's dire event.

We chatted about nothing important as I observed her administer the breathing treatment and physiotherapy and ready Heather for bed. She correctly positioned the small plastic square pads of the cardiorespiratory alarm on a foam belt and wrapped it round Heather's chest.

Melissa smoothed Heather's nightgown and tucked a soft blanket around the quiet child. She stretched back the thin, green elastic strap of the clear plastic trach mask and eased the mask down into place over the trach tube. Powering up the mist-producing compressor, its motor sounded like acorns rolling across a tin roof. It moistened the air that Heather inhaled via the mask. Heather reposed, ready for bed without any fuss.

Serving as an audible notice of secretions pooling in the trach, the resonance of loud gurgling breaths jarred Jim and me awake. Knowing they could harden and plug the trach frightened us. Sounds of Melissa's use of the suction machine gave clues to her skill. Hearing Heather's easy breathing resume permitted us to doze off. When a Jamaican lullaby roused me from sporadic sleep, I burrowed into the covers, confident that Melissa would love our baby.

All the world shone new to Heather—raindrops, dancing butterflies, and outdoor swings. Jim and I planned to immerse her in an atmosphere of love, one that expected recovery; but if she didn't improve, we'd adore her just as she was, wouldn't we?

"Sunshine will do her good—might even cure her. She sure didn't get any rays in the hospital," Jim said in jest, but half-serious.

With Heather in his arms, he knelt on the dew-laden grass next to a hovering dragonfly. Jim shifted her to a standing position and kept hold of her sides. She refused to bear weight. Her legs dangled, knees bent, bare feet hovering, not touching the grass. By accident she kicked out until her dainty toes brushed the green blades, but her feet recoiled as if touching fire. Jim relocated the standing lesson to a spot of sun-dried earth. Her fidgety toes pressed into the sandy soil made her jump faster than a cricket.

"Shoot!" Jim said, his standard response to any minor unexpected happening. "Sneakers may help," he surmised, and looked up smiling. He asked Jamie to go rummage up a pair.

Daddy Jim slipped Heather's feet into light pink athletic shoes and adjusted the laces. Jamie and Tony coached words of encouragement. Body held, feet covered, little Heather took short prancing steps. Satin hair ribbons and wispy chestnut bangs fluttered, her eyebrows shifted a trifle. The drooping corners of her mouth upturned a speck.

Jim loosened his hold, and Heather balanced solo, before toppling onto her diapered bottom. Now sitting, Heather shifted her gaze and studied big sister's cartwheels with intense focus. Mischievous Tony lost interest and poked a stick at an anthill.

Sherry from across the street walked over. "Wait a minute. Something's changed in how you clothe your daughters," she said, chuckling. "I don't recall Jamie wearing fancy outfits. Bet you'll regret frilly dresses, when teenage Heather insists on expensive attire."

"Ah maybe so, too funny," I replied. "All the dazzle camouflages her slightly odd and dusky appearance."

"Come on over, your parents too. My boys love Heather. They've started jabbering about wanting a sister," Sherry said. Tony capered ahead to join his buddies.

Once inside, the freckle-faced, red-haired brothers emptied their toy box, offering Heather each item. "Truck," said Tom with an earnest expression. "Fish," he offered next. "Helicopter, look how it spins," he said, as he flicked the rotor.

Heather worked silent magic, drawing all closer. Inspired, Sam lifted her onto the piano bench. He grinned his giant twinkling smile as he took her hand in his, and together they plunked the keys in a simple melody. Heather's nose wrinkled a trifle in acknowledgement.

"I think she's smart," my mom piped up, summarizing recent observations. "Yet I worry about her lack of expression."

"She'll be fine, Mom," I replied. "Really she will. I know it."

Home again to administer Heather's treatments. Preparation and clean-up claimed sixty minutes every four hours around the clock. Tossing in ordinary household and family chores tilted Jim and me into exhaustion.

To prepare the breathing treatment, Jim squirted a half cc of albuterol (to open the airways) and three cc of saline into a hard plastic bubble that unscrewed in the middle. He toggled on the nebulizer. The machine blew air via a tubing into the chamber of albuterol solution transforming it into a medicated vapor that Heather would breathe for ten minutes.

One-quarter hour of vibratory chest physiotherapy followed. Jim laid Heather tummy-down across his pillow-cushioned knees and clapped and jiggled her back with a gentle cupped hand. Rolling her over, he repeated the percussions on her chest and each side to loosen the sticky secretions inside her lungs. Otherwise mucous clogged her small airways, trapping stale air.

Sometimes children voiced concern about the vaporized "smoke" and "hitting." Individual sessions on the doubters dispersed their fears as each discovered it felt rather pleasant, like a back massage.

Coughing and more coughing ensued as the treatment progressed. Mucous gurgled and bubbled into her trach. Jim grasped a slender, hollow, red-rubber catheter and gently inserted and suctioned her trach tube and trachea to augment her ineffective efforts at ridding the mucous. Never did she fight the intrusions to her body, exhibiting only placid acceptance even when the catheter touched the delicate mucosa of her natural airways.

Nourishment followed physiotherapy so she'd not be jiggled on a full stomach. Jim poured baby formula into the refillable two-ounce holding syringe, and it dripped down tubing and through the gastrostomy button into her stomach. Rapidity of flow depended on gravity and how high we held the syringe. Afterward we put her down for a nap in her crib.

To miss hearing an alarm would mean death. As a precaution, an extension wire snaked down the hall to sound an additional alarm that we could position close to whatever we were doing. To roam a tad farther, such as to get the mail or empty the trash or do laundry in the garage, we utilized a two-part baby monitor. Resembling a walkie-talkie, it functioned as an eavesdropper for hearing alarms and the sounds of Heather's breathing. If both were quiet, hearing the background noise of the compressor assured us of the monitor's effective transmission.

Laura and Melissa were superb nurses. Jim called the nursing agency and requested that they divvy up the seven nights and work a set schedule. No others, especially not that evil one, Jim stipulated. The manager complied, yet made a strong plea for considering the services of a day nurse, one who had worked with Heather at the Wilsons' home.

"Our life is a circus. No more additions." Jim refuted the idea.

"Your wife could run errands without lugging Heather and her equipment along." The man pointed out a litany of additional advantages.

"Being toted around with mom is a normal part of childhood," Jim rebutted.

"Please consider letting Betsey come once? She's despondent about losing touch."

"Well, maybe," Jim acquiesced. "Let me ask Ann which day is best."

That second weekend of Heather's homecoming, my folks returned. Jamie was playing with Heather on a blanket spread beneath a mimosa when they arrived. "How are my two granddaughters?" Mom asked.

After supper Dad dumped out the contents of a brown paper sack on our dining table, making it obvious what had been worrying him. "Now Heather's trach will never fall out," he guaranteed. Tinkering in his workshop he'd conceived a half-dozen different designs for foolproof ties. Father- and son-in-law carefully reviewed proposed and existing designs.

Little Heather tilted her head to better see what Granddad was concocting next. A pair of cushioned stainless-steel ones wrapped almost twice around her neck. "Smaller than I thought," Dad said with unusual seriousness.

"Only a blow torch could get those off. You sure can tell Granddad's an engineer." Jamie laughed.

"Steel won't fail, but impossible to cut if there's an urgent need to pull out a plugged trach," Jim explained.

Despite advantages to Dad's sturdier models, we concluded that cloth ties seemed safest if secured properly as twill can be cut in a flash. Scissors and an extra trach were always in reach in my purse, taped to the crib, and stashed in the panic kits—one kept on the dresser and another in the emergency bag. As we'd experienced, cloth ties have drawbacks. Knots can fray or fail or be tied incorrectly. Twill stretches, and with the slack, a trach can fall out and hang like a pendant on a necklace. Velcro—little hands of the child or a friend can unfasten them anytime.

Mom and Dad took Heather outside to the grape arbor. In a baby swing, pale Heather swayed beneath the gnarled vines. My young-looking parents vied for attention. Dad removed his floppy hat and placed it atop the quiet child's head and told stories of the ocean. Mom sang songs.

Inside again, Mom sat on the couch reading the children storybooks and then made a brilliant suggestion. "Maybe if Tony drinks from a bottle, Heather would mimic him." Tony balked at first. She persuaded him to let her cradle him in her arms like a baby, but he wiggled out in protest, trudged around the couch, stopping beside Heather.

"Don't anyone tell my friends, ever," three-year-old Tony insisted. "Watch big brother," he said, standing close. He sucked milk out of the bottle, and then offered it to his new baby sister. After a couple of go-rounds, Heather let Tony place the bottle in her mouth. "Good girl," he said, a smile plumping his chubby cheeks. "You can do it," he encouraged again and again. We crossed our fingers, hoping she wouldn't choke. Heather swallowed two ounces. "Yeah, you did it," Tony cheered. The remaining milk we poured into the holding syringe and dripped it into her buttoned stomach.

All daytime tube feedings were phased out over the next week. Instead Heather drank milk from a bottle, stopping when she wanted, freely determining how much formula ended up in her tummy. After two more weeks we eliminated all nighttime tube feedings without replacing them with any bottles. With the consumption of oral nourishment, the ugly sucking-in-the-lips stopped, and she no longer drooled. Confidence reigned that she'd make up the lost calories during the day, though we'd keep a close tab on her weight.

Medical care swallowed up all hours of the day. I cut back to working only one day on the weekend. We threw out false pride and took advantage of an offer of discounted shopping at the local food bank. Humbled, we sought refuge at our church and prayed for God's strength and guidance.

Jamie played sisterly games. "Sit down, stand up, turn yourself around," Jamie chanted as she moved Heather through the motions. Animal imitations came next. Jamie shook Heather's fists and drummed her chest, while making gorilla noises. Heather scrunched her nose. Jim hooted like an owl, and I squished my lips and moved them like a fish.

Out back, Jim deposited Heather into our oversized knotted-rope hammock. Fresh young leaves sprouted from the overhead tree branches. A flock of blackbirds took flight, swirling in the crisp air. Numerous robins hopped about, pecking through dry leaves to the ground, adding their calls and commotion to a day of celebrating life.

Neighborhood kids raced into the back yard, and about six clambered in with Heather. Jamie set to pushing the loaded hammock-cocoon, almost ready to burst loose its load of squirming, giggling youngsters. Chris Little, the most boisterous of the bunch, championed imaginative quests of pretending to be monkeys escaping predators, or pirates in a leaky vessel surrounded by snapping alligators.

Neither car seemed big enough to carry the family and medical equipment, or in an emergency to perform resuscitation. Jim scanned the newspaper's classified section and tapped an ad that intrigued him. A full-size van was for sale way out in Keystone Heights. He took the scenic route and called me almost breathless with anticipation. "By the posh appearance of the lakefront home and its landscaping, the Ford will be a cream puff. Okay if I make the decision without you?" he asked.

The next day a friend gave him a ride back, and Jim drove home the six-year-old top-of-the-line vehicle equipped with all the bells and whistles. The van purchase necessitated the bittersweet sale of Jim's orange '72 VW Bug. He'd owned it for seventeen years, three years longer than he had known me. A college student purchased it and seemed quite smitten despite the car's dents and missing right rear fender. The young man handed us cash.

"Shoot!" Jim said, as the VW disappeared from view.

"What?" I asked.

"The broken gas gauge," Jim said. "I forgot to tell him."

"Whoops, dang it. I haven't his phone number," I replied.

Jim offered an odd reassurance. "After a few stalls, he'll figure it out, that the tank goes empty at the half-full mark."

The afternoon of the baby shower, in deference to the guests, Mark and Celeste banished their two family dogs to the backyard. Choo-Choo, a German shepherd mix, whimpered, nose pressed imploringly to a windowpane. They referred to him as the Heather-dog, as he too had been rescued from a hopeless future. Bestowed tongue-in cheek, Choo-Choo's name was a reminder of the unfortunate truth: he'd been hit by a train.

Heather wore an early present, a white ruffled blouse with pink bows on the sleeves and matching soft canvas overalls. Jamie's skirt swirled as she spun around. Tony sported a favorite muscle shirt.

Guests milled about a lace-covered table laden with pastry, muffins, and raspberry punch.

"A toast to Heather and her burgeoning health and the beauty of an unfolding miracle." Celeste clinked her coffee cup to mine and Maria's. Jamie sat near to the tower of gifts with Heather on her lap. Both watched as I opened the presents. That wonderful celebration made formal the community's welcoming of our new (hopefully forever, not temporary) daughter, and we all rejoiced with one heart.

The give her a chance day-nurse came the next day. With a plethora of visitors, no longer did Jim and I tidy the house for anyone, not new or established nurses, suppliers, social workers, friends, or family. All got it as it happened to be—cluttered, immaculate, dirty, or messy.

Betsey's straight dark hair hung half-way down her back. She wore jeans and slung a canvas-pack over her shoulder. "Hello, honey. I missed you," she said to Heather. Next she turned her attention to Tony. "And what's your name?" She eased her pack down, sat cross-legged on the floor. Betsey pulled out a mix of stuffed animals and trucks and books and toys and set about entertaining all three children. Jamie and Heather looked cute in their matching sweatshirts.

"Okay if I go outside and mow the yard?" I asked. She nodded, and I felt like a kid let out for recess.

The day went well, so I asked her to please come every Tuesday.

"I'd love to," she answered.

"In the morning, I'll volunteer in Jamie's classroom. Per policy I know already that I can only leave Heather in your care. My friend Celeste will watch Tony." Betsey would stay on until Jim arrived home. A godsend, I could run errands, exercise, and spend after-school time with Jamie and Tony without the distraction of complicated Heather.

Heather's muteness affected me in an unexpected way. Sometimes she felt borrowed. She lived so close to death. It was nothing but the truth, I confided in my sister. "When forming a mental picture of her, she seems more a mirage than someone real. Instead of thinking about a person's physical form, it seems that I create images of people more through their words and gestures." For Heather the former was impossible, and she'd barely developed the latter.

"Heather is as real to you as a person gets." Kristin discounted the whole notion.

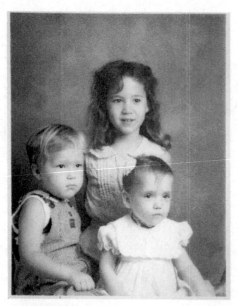

Young Tony, Jamie, and Heather Giganti

CHAPTER 13] SMOKE-OUT

Heather didn't move her fingers. We thought it probable that she'd figure out how. Verbal language was truly physically impossible. Babies learn to talk by hearing their family speak, so we figured Heather would learn the language of fingers and hands by observing our family communicate that way. *Signing Exact English*: the book traveled with us everywhere. Alphabetically, words and their corresponding signs were depicted by line drawings of hand motions and facial expression.

Feeding the ducks at the park, we sat down at a picnic table. Jamie looked up some animal signs. An aggressive goose stuck its clacking bill close, and Tony skedaddled up the bench onto the tabletop. Two other children pranced over with their mothers. The language of hands provided instant entertainment. All seemed drawn to its creative and humorous interpretation of what it depicted.

"How are we to keep up with her need for signed words?" Jim asked. Forming hand movements seemed easy, but remembering the immense number seemed about as feasible as outracing an avalanche. Photocopies of ten important signs, like mom, dad, more, please, thank you, and drink, were placed in strategic places. The four of us agreed to simultaneously sign the words every time we spoke them.

Signing words with my fingers in public places definitely shot my preference to fade into the crowd. We already garnered attention because of Heather's conspicuously noisy neck breathing. One advantage was the ability to silently scold the kids by the gestures, *No* or *I will spank your bottom,* from nearby or afar.

Unlike the menace they posed in the hospital, no vicious germs lingered in the shadows of our home. Every other day Jim and I super-cleaned certain medical supplies. We did the tasks, instead of delegating them, as we had more at stake than the nurses on duty. Poorly cleaned, contaminated equipment could inoculate Heather's lungs with threatening disease.

All tubing, masks, chambers, and storage items were soaked in a special solution to kill respiratory bacteria and viruses. Electric and battery-powered equipment was wiped down with the same.

Reusable catheters required ten minutes of boiling. A "clean" procedure, not sterile, but it was good enough. Simmering in a pot of water, the red rubber suction catheters coiled up among themselves like odd-shaped eels.

"Jim, can't I please take over boiling them?" Nurse Laura urged.

"No, thanks," he said. The offer held no appeal.

"It is almost midnight. Surely you are fatigued. At least I can relieve you of this one chore," the good-natured woman stressed, her face puckering into a knowing frown.

"Ah, don't worry about it." Jim shrugged off the idea.

"Please," she insisted.

Jim wearily gave in and passed over the tongs. She set to work stirring the steaming mix, then plucking out the catheters and laying them on the drying towel. I kept her company. When finished, we looked in on our little champion fight-for-life girl.

"She's a charmer," Nurse Laura said as she tenderly touched Heather's pale cheek. "I don't know how she does it, can't say a word yet steals the heart of anyone who cares for her. Maybe it's having to pay close attention. Her expressions are tenuous, almost invisible."

"They're not subtle when you are her mama," I said, looking down at my sweet bundle.

"So far her eyes have not opened even a smidgeon during the nighttime respiratory treatments and physiotherapy. It is tempting to rouse her and play," Laura said.

"What? Now don't go and spoil her," I responded, scowling in jest. "Sleeping through the night is a blessing. Jamie and Tony always sprang out of bed as if it were a hot potato."

In the mornings, Laura would offer Heather colorful toys. Arms hanging limp, Heather made no attempts to grasp any of them. Laura placed a rattle in Heather's hand, layering her own hand on top. She moved hand and rattle through a variety of shakes. Heather's passive visage persisted.

Monthly pre-surgery clinic came around too fast. A double-stroller made getting around easier; Heather in the front seat, her equipment in the back. In the waiting area, I befriended a woman whose little daughter had a trach, but the child could talk! How stupendous to hear the child's hushed voice. A little older than Heather, Samantha talked in whispery words by using a Passy-Muir® speaking valve. She scooted closer to Heather on the bench seat and read aloud a book by Dr. Seuss.

Information about the public school system gave me one of those feel-sick-to-my-stomach moments. "Children with tracheotomies aren't allowed in the regular classrooms," Samantha's mother disclosed.

"Disheartening. I hadn't given it any thought. Limiting Heather's curriculum to special education classes might hinder her potential. Separate is not equal," I spoke softly. More hurdles, guess they'd never stop.

"Private school may be an option, if Heather ever becomes able to talk," she said. "A local one accepted Samantha. The principal is enthusiastic and diligent. He had several teachers undergo training in tracheotomy care. Pivotal to his decision was Samantha's good lungs and health. She can talk, so she can tell the teachers whenever she needs suctioning or whether something is wrong."

"Maybe we can sidestep this dismal issue if Heather gets her tracheotomy out. The surgeon is convinced monthly bronchoscopic dilations will eliminate the scarring and that Heather will talk, even if the frailness of her lungs thwarts removing the trach." I decided to postpone thinking about school until necessary.

The nurse called Heather's name.

I told the surgeon the wonderful news that Heather took all nourishment by mouth. No weight loss. She'd even gained a pound. "When is the soonest the feeding hole in her stomach can be closed?" I asked.

"In a year," the surgeon answered.

"That is way too long." I disagreed.

"A conservative approach is best. What if she becomes ill and refuses to drink?" he asked.

"She'd get intravenous fluids like anybody else," I replied.

"But she doesn't eat food; she only drinks formula," he rebutted. "Maybe in six months the g-button can be removed if there are no problems. I wouldn't want to turn right around and perform surgery to create another one."

Jim took a bright red marker and circled the target date on the kitchen calendar.

A helpless newborn and an inquisitive two-year-old all wrapped up in one package was a good description of Heather at that time. Her whirlwind progress and accomplishments toward learning what she'd missed and catching up to age-appropriate skills made Jim and me dizzy. How drastically things could change in six weeks amazed us.

Metamorphosis of attitude—Heather's care wasn't frightening! It was as routine as brushing our teeth and as automatic as the sun's rising, just part of an ordinary day. If a palm reader had foretold such a change would come to pass, Jim and I would have scoffed at the idea.

In for some smooth sailing, we thought, until one night at 4:18 a.m.

"Ann. Jim," Nurse Laura knocked lightly on our door. "There's a problem," she put forth hesitantly.

A whiff of acrid smoke burned my nose, eyes, and lungs. "No fire. I scorched the suction catheters. All the water boiled away in the pot on the stove." The small mound of melted rubber billowed forth voluminous fumes that engulfed the hallway.

"Jim, grab Tony; I'll get the girls!" We slammed bedroom doors behind us to keep out the noxious gases and gathered the children and Heather's emergency equipment and rushed all of us outside into the fresh night air. We deposited all three children into the oversized hammock and wrapped them in a comforter, where they snuggled sleepily.

The catastrophe was limited to the pot. Any flames had dissipated. We hadn't any need to call the fire department. It was mind boggling how much stinky fumes a pan of melting rubber created. A distraught Laura faltered out her explanation. "I had the burner turned to high and went back to keep an eye on Heather. I started reading my book and plain forgot."

The two dozen red rubber catheters would not have filled a soup bowl, yet the awful stench left no crevice of our home untouched. The whitish smoke deposited a colorless residue everywhere. If it had been black, all would have been ruined. The whole of that awful day was spent trying to air out the house. We finally acknowledged defeat. After completing the arduous task of packing up Heather's supplies, we retreated to a motel. Reassembling her medical equipment to make the room with two double beds have the capability of a PICU left us in a state of exhaustion.

The nursing home-health agency contracted with professionals for the clean-up.

"Why had none of the four smoke alarms gone off?" Jim asked the foreman.

"They all buzzed when we pumped in the neutralizing vapor," the foreman replied. "The smoke that rubber catheters produce is not common in house fires. It won't set off standard home smoke alarms; you need a different specialized rating."

Jim and I thanked God for our safety. The children thought it was great fun, watching TV in the cramped motel room, eating delivered pizza, and swimming in the pool.

"Take me off the case," volunteered the errant nurse when she checked on us.

"No. We'll learn together," Jim replied, "but no tending to Heather in this small room. There's no space." We stayed at a hotel for three days while huge fans and special chemicals blew through the house like a November gale; the bad odor detectable blocks away.

An unexpected boon came from the fireless fire. Courage in our ability to pack up Heather and her many supplies and safely provide overnight care rooted in as a continuing possibility. Perhaps we could do without the nurses. We'd have to obtain permission, as Heather was officially—a temporary, foster child.

We still mummy-wrapped her every day to install fresh ties and once a week to swap out to a clean trach. Eight-year-old Jamie could expertly perform all of Heather's nursing care, including assisting with the weekly trach changes and daily fresh ties.

Heather's need for nighttime suctioning decreased, and we tried eliminating routine breathing treatments between midnight and six in the morning. Baby girl napped a long spell each afternoon without fuss; otherwise she tired and struggled more in her efforts to breathe.

Illness took hold of Heather a few days before the next scheduled bronchoscopy. She looked as floppy and blue tinged as that first time Jim met her. Antibiotics, frequent breathing treatments, and a continuous humidifying mist kept her lungs tenuously working.

Confidence in our ability to care for her stemmed from knowing we possessed the same ammunition as a hospital—topped off by the fairy dust of tender love bestowed in her own home. Fear tempted us to give her fluids through the gastrostomy. But slow and determined, Heather drank the entire contents of her milk bottles as Jim or I or one of the nurses rocked her. After a week's vigil, Heather rallied. The illness had us put the no-nurses idea on the back burner.

Heather had appointments at preoperative clinic for a chest x-ray and labs. Most Medicaid doctor appointments were time-consuming, all day affairs. There was no incentive for courtesy and expedience as we had no choice to go elsewhere. As though undercover investigators, I witnessed the sometimes excellent, but often poor treatment of the medically needy.

Another waiting mom began chatting with me. "Keep meticulous records," she cautioned. "Someone who lacks understanding of your daughter's health problems might anonymously call HRS with allegations of abuse. Proof of adequate care will ward off heartbreak. Log progress, appointments, medications, and take photographs."

"Thanks for the advice. I've heard distressing stories."

Tony grabbed lollipops from the clinic's basket and offered one to Heather. She stuck a cherry one inside her mouth! Glory be did she look cute eating candy like any other child!

A phlebotomist stuck her vein for a few vials of blood. Vigorous nonvocal crying bubbled up copious gurgles. I toggled on the portable suction machine and gently inserted a red rubber catheter to clear the trach tube.

At radiology the X-ray tech strapped Heather into a plastic restraining "space suit" and shot several chest films. The images showed right-upper-lobe collapse and fuzzy scarring and air-trapping, all chronic conditions for her. We hand-carried the films to an anesthesiologist, and after he cleared her for surgery, we left for home.

Heather's weekly appointments included occupational and physical therapy. In a play room with tumbling mats, a therapist exercised Heather with the aid of balls. Some were large enough to stretch her over, others small to strengthen fingers. College students observed through a one-way mirror as a part of their studies.

Speech—the third weekly therapy—reinforced Heather's budding venture into communication by further introducing the sign language of the deaf. Her therapist blew puffs of air through a soapy wand. Glistening bubbles popped on Heather's nose. The therapist formed the word *bubble* with her free hand. Heather's eyes showed pleasure, though her fingers remained immobile.

Each evening, Jamie snatched Heather up, and they'd sit together in the middle of the twin bed. Next, Jamie stood on top of the covers and jumped as easily as if it were a trampoline, mattress-bouncing Heather. Both girls giggled—Jamie out loud and Heather silently. With great agility, Jamie would catch hold of her little sister, and they'd flop down on the carpet to play the daily game of "stand up, sit down," with Jamie assisting Heather until at last Heather could stand, balanced on her own. "Good girl, Heather!" Jamie cheered. "I knew you could do it."

Heather's body weight continued to increase without the tube feedings. Nurse Laura began tempting her with baby food. Heather pursed her lips and knitted her brow. The only nourishment Heather would accept was formula from a bottle, which now that her arms were stronger, she preferred to hold by herself.

Tony took over the offering of tastes of pureed fruit. "Watch big brother," he coaxed while making funny faces and spouting amusing comments as good as any comedian's. One day he managed to sneak in a bit of peach. She smacked and gummed, not spitting it out, ultimately swallowing it. Using sweetness to entice her learning to eat, cookies came next. Healthful foods we would introduce in their own time. No need to push.

My brother, Mike, invited us over for grilled chicken. April's sunny weather had warmed up the community pool at his condominium. Mike challenged me to a freestyle swim race. I was winning, but stopped suddenly at the sight of a plummeting bat pivoting to skim across the surface. The little creature flitted upward and circled before descending again to resume his thirst-quenching flight.

"Oh, him," Mike said. "He joins me whenever I swim near dusk."

Everyone toweled off and went inside. Clutching the arm of a chair, Heather crawled up to a stand. Jamie jangled a bunch of keys, enticing her to toddle a short distance. Again and again she chanced a step, determined to acquire the prize. Success! She walked five or six steps, eyes sparkling, but no other muscles in her face moved. She breathed harder, and her trach sounded a cadence of happy gurgles that might have bothered a stranger, but we'd grown accustomed to it.

Maybe just maybe, one day she'd get the trach out and become physically able to talk. Maybe just maybe, she'd become our forever daughter. And maybe, Jim and I could manage her care without having nurses in our home.

Life was the best it had ever been. Perhaps it was Heather who immersed us in an envelope of love, not the other way around.

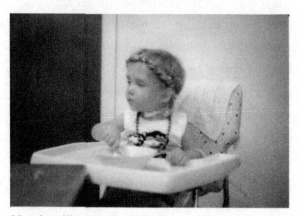

Heather likes her bangles.

CHAPTER 14] MORE CLASSES

Legally, Heather could not become our forever-and-ever daughter until we attended the required series of adoption classes. At any time, HRS powers-that-be could yank Heather from us and place her with a different family, already licensed for adoption. No one knew when the classes would be offered.

With Heather's improving mobility, physical and occupational therapy appointments went out the window. Her new antic sealed our belief that she was brilliant. Heather placed a pair of Jim's shoes at his feet then scuttled the hallway and dropped sneakers by Jamie. She raced off again to bring Tony his tennis shoes. One more excursion and she returned with her own shoes and mine. She tugged each of us one at a time toward the front door. Though she'd not yet signed a single word, she'd pantomimed her first sentence: "Let's go somewhere as a family—now!" How canny that she noticed we only wore shoes when leaving for an outing.

Lingering for a moment in our garden, Jamie and Tony plucked some ripening blueberries and ate them just as fast, spitting out the occasional sour one. A wondrous sense of new horizons accompanied us on our walk along the wooded trail to my brother's townhome.

"Come see my new saltwater fish," Mike invited when we reached there. The kids peered at a pair of yellow tangs swimming among the conch shells. A clown fish wriggled deep into a purple-tipped anemone. Banded cleaner shrimps clambered over sea urchin spikes.

"Let's play bear trap, Uncle Mike!" the kids begged. Our dad had dreamed up the game of lazy-father tag. Now Mike acted the role of the hungry grizzly. He sprawled on the floor while Jamie, Tony, and Heather dashed around him while trying to avoid getting captured. "Gotcha," Michael growled, snagging Heather with his paw.

Heather bloomed with vibrant giggles, seen but not heard. Jamie and Tony jabbed with their fists, scampering away while Heather wiggled and twisted to no avail. She remained ensnared until Michael Bear feigned sleep, pretend-snoring in raspy grumbles. His paws went limp. Heather slipped away to freedom, then resumed the game.

Mike's medical school graduation was set for May 26. Next he'd go to Nashville for a year of general surgery.

"Everyone is coming," Mike said. "Both grandmas, Mark and Jeanette, Kristin and Chuck. Out-of-towners and locals are staying at the Gainesville Hilton," he said.

"Reserve a suite for us, assuming we can obtain permission from HRS," Jim said.

"Grandmother Pat wants to bunk with your family. She's eager to meet Heather," Mike said.

A desire to work in health care had been sparked by stories told by Mom's parents, who were a nurse and doctor team. All Irish, Granddaddy Doctor fought boxing matches and won poker games to earn money for medical school. They started out delivering babies in 1928, one year before the Depression. "Times were hard. Families often paid us in chickens," Grandmother Pat said. If no patients waited in their humble office, he'd shoot billiards in the adjacent pool hall until one showed up.

In the small farming town of McCune, Kansas, mothers gave birth in the comfort of their homes, usually reposed on the kitchen table. Often the family dog lay underneath. Rubber sheeting funneled birth water into a bucket. The father stayed with his wife or busied himself with chores, depending on his temperament.

Even in tough times, my grandparents liked to dress in the latest styles. It got them into notorious trouble once because of mistaken identities. Photographs show a petite woman, quite the looker, about five feet two, decked out in a fitted dress, heels, and a tilted cloche. Granddaddy was six feet tall and muscular. He wore a tailored suit, and on his head, a wool fedora, and always had a lit Camel cigarette.

Farm homes were great distances apart. Often they borrowed a vehicle and drove separately in case Doctor was needed elsewhere. Based on their travel, Model A Ford, fashion, and preferred cigarettes, vigilante detectives concluded the couple were the notorious gangsters, Bonnie and Clyde, who had a hide-out in nearby Joplin, Missouri.

All aiming their Tommy sub-machine rifles, government agents piled inside and on the hood of an unmarked police vehicle and forced Grandmother to swerve off the road. "'Bonnie,' they called out to me. One agent realized their mistake, and the posse screeched away from a most ominous blunder," Grandmother said, when recalling the incident.

HRS and the medical caseworker granted approval for the family weekend. Next I posed the question that had begun brewing with the smoke-out. "If caring for Heather graduation weekend goes well, can we permanently go without in-home nurses?"

"I'll ask the doctors, but I can't predict what they'll say," the nurse specialist answered.

"Tell them we crafted a jingle-bell bracelet so she can shake it noisily to beckon our attention." The call-your-parent idea amused her, and she promised to phone when she had an answer.

Too soon, it was again time for her monthly bronchoscopy. Wake-up alarm chimed at 6:00 a.m. At the hospital, there was no dedicated waiting room for children undergoing an operation. A few chairs in a corner of the large visitors' lobby located next to the main entrance were reserved for the purpose. Bob, the teaching nurse, walked through the glass doors, and I waved.

"Heather looks good." He tugged at his beard. "You and Jim are nuts, but good nuts."

"You believe in these children too," I chided, holding his gaze.

"Well yes, but I don't know if I'd go so far as to take one home," he answered.

Bronchoscopic dilation surgery doesn't take long, and I was soon at her cribside in the PICU. Heather blinked at me through groggy eyes. I suctioned blood-streaked mucous, going no deeper than the length of the trach tube. Intuitively Jim and I had begun stopping short of contacting the delicate mucosa of her natural airway. She no longer ignored intrusions to her body, and deeper suctioning made her cough painfully. Our technique opposed what the instructors taught in nursing school: they had us suction deep into the trachea until the catheter could pass no further.

I tended her, oblivious to the other children in the unit. I reviewed the physician's post-op orders and was disheartened to find tube feedings among them despite my spoken and written update. "Please get this error corrected," I insisted. "Heather gets her nourishment from bottles and baby food now. She'll get upset if a tube feeding appears." An oversight or hadn't the doctor believed me?

A nurse moved Heather to my arms. Baby Girl busied herself picking the adhesive visitor's tag off my blouse. An overnight hospital stay with observation in the PICU for complications was standard post-operative care for trach kids. Lungs can get punctured from surgical manipulations and thus collapse. Stretching of scar tissue by dilating rods scrapes the delicate mucosa. The resultant abrasions always generated abundant bloody secretions. Extra vigilance prevented and alleviated scary plugs in her tracheotomy tube that would block her breathing.

The bronchoscopic surgeon didn't answer when I asked whether he'd dilated the scarring enough for Heather to talk. "Any chance of spacing the bronchs farther apart?" I asked, emphasizing that it took her ten days to recuperate.

"Not any time soon," the surgeon answered.

"How long will monthly dilations be necessary?" I asked.

"Until she's six years old," he answered.

My disappointment showed in vivid colors. It meant she'd still have the trach when she was to begin kindergarten.

Jim relieved me when he got off work and remained at her cribside until she fell asleep. Hospital policy wouldn't allow us to stay with her overnight. We weren't too worried about her missing us. She always seemed to sleep through until morning, and I'd return early before she awakened, and then bring her home.

A month passed, and she underwent another bronchoscopy with dilation. After the procedure, the sight of her in PICU shocked me. They'd tied her hands to the bed, because she was in a bed, not a crib. Usually they contained her in a "cage crib"—a mattress fully enclosed by side rails tall enough to meet its barred ceiling. Sobbing, she fought the restraints. Silent crying induced copious gurgles that almost roared with the rushing of her pressured breathing.

Gentle suctioning cleared the trach of the thick noisy mucous. I undid the knots to free her, and snugged my child close. Calming down, she began picking off my stick-on visitor's tag. Anytime anyone in blue scrubs neared, Heather squeezed me tight and bawled. A half-hour later a nurse flagged my attention. "You have to leave, Mrs. Giganti. It's shift change."

I beseeched her to make an exception. "Heather can't make any noise when she cries. She can't talk or form signed words with her fingers. Besides, I am a nurse. I work here in labor and delivery."

The stern nurse refused to budge. "It's the rule," she repeated like a parrot, her words echoing.

"She'll tumble right over the six-inch siderails on this bed and fall to the floor. At home she sleeps in a baby crib." I insisted that she have one. Finding it would take hours, I thought, eliminating the quandary. Wrong. The insensitive nurse must have been wearing roller skates. She returned with a fully enclosed crib and moved Heather into it.

There was no spare trach in the room, so I handed the nurse one from my purse and left the unit blinded by tears. I might have fussed more but was afraid. HRS adoptions were political, and there were more doors to unlock. I hurried downstairs, out the main door, and walked two brisk laps around the hospital in sweltering heat before phoning Jim, Mike, and Celeste in hopes of regaining my composure.

Memories of Maria's experience surfaced. Limitations on parental visitation made no sense. A parent caring for a child reduces a nurse's workload. Professed concerns about confidentiality can be overcome by conducting staff reports in a conference room instead of at the bedside.

Still sniffling my way back to PICU, I detoured to labor and delivery and talked to one of my friends there. I shuffled back to Heather's side, looking only at her, avoiding contact with any nurse. Late that evening the surgeon stopped by.

"Can't my husband or I stay with Heather tonight?" I asked, politely expressing my view that sequestering her from family was unmerited.

"No," he said, but offered a future solution. "On the general pediatric floor there's a ward room equipped with cardiorespiratory monitoring. Parents may stay with their child around the clock. Heather can go there for post-op observation next time."

Good news came our way via the medical caseworker. The no-nurse request scored a home run, unanimous agreement after our handling of the smoke incident.

"When can we inform the nurses that they're no longer needed?" I asked.

"Today."

"Shouldn't they receive two-weeks notice?"

"It's entirely your decision."

I confirmed that we'd keep Betsey coming one day a week.

The jangling bells flopped as a call-your-parent device. Heather moved around too much, and they cling-clanged constantly."

Jim's new brainstorm was mounting a bike horn on the crib rail. Tony blared the horn, and then coaxed Heather. He guided her through the hand motion to sound the horn. She proceeded to attempt doing it 'all by herself,' but didn't have the strength. Maybe success would come in the near future.

Two weeks passed. Bidding farewell to Laura and Melissa felt bittersweet. We'd grown quite fond of them. Not that the kids considered no night-nurses an improvement, to them their presence was like having Grandma over for unending slumber parties.

"Heather will be missed." Laura's eyes welled with tears on her last morning. She hugged us and said, "Your family is the nicest folks I've ever worked for."

Newfound privacy nudged the relaxation quotient up several notches. Our first night alone felt like we'd popped a cork out of a champagne bottle, and we effervesced with mirth. "No more late knocks on the door; no having to socialize when you'd rather be snoozing." Jim recited a chronicle of advantages. "More time for romance." He winked.

"No outside company at breakfast time," I chimed in.

"Back in my own bed!" Jamie exclaimed. Both girls clambered up on top of the mattress. Holding hands, they began jumping. Plopping down on top of the orange comforter, they took a short break from the hopping. To our great surprise, Heather extended her left hand, palm up. With her right index and middle fingers bending at the knuckles, she repeatedly bounced them off her left palm—the sign for *jump*.

"I taught it to her," Jamie beamed.

Heather formed additional signs in rapid succession: *mom, dad, candy, more,* and *dollar* (more money to buy chocolates). At last her fingers had enough strength to make the movements her mind had been absorbing. Happiness shined in her slightly crinkled eyes and subtle movements of her lips, overcoming the immobile mask of the rest of her face.

In the wee hours of the morning, doubts pecked at Jim about having no nurse, and he nudged me. "What if the alarms fail or we don't waken fast enough? One of us should be closer to Heather, but Jamie shouldn't get booted out of her bed." Going to the garage, he retrieved a sleeping bag and unrolled it on the floor of the girls' room. "If her breathing goes wrong, I'll hear it and tend to it before the situation deteriorates enough to trigger any alarms."

"Great idea, safer," I said, and hugged my caring Jim. At least the girls would have a more normal routine. They wouldn't really be aware he slept there on the floor. He went to bed after they did and wakened before.

"I'd take a turn on floor duty, but I can't," I said. Every second of the day I tuned in to Heather's breathing and had to turn off at some point.

We were so eager to finalize the adoption. Cindy Smith wanted to wrap things up as much as we did. "Another county is offering the adoption course series. If you don't mind the drive, it would meet our requirement," she suggested.

"When does it begin?" I asked trying to sound nonchalant.

"Next week," she replied. "Can you make it?"

"Of course, most certainly."

Marlene, an occupational therapy student, would babysit for Jamie and Tony on class nights. Level-headed Betsey agreed to work extra hours and care for Heather.

In sheer delight, voiceless Heather greeted Betsey with a self-discovered and most unusual way of claiming attention. Heather would lower her chin, pressing it against her neck and pinching off the trach tube's opening. Then she forcefully exhaled until some air squeaked through the tightly touching skin of chin and neck to sound the loud blast of a trumpeting elephant, with following sputters. On class nights, all three children enjoyed dedicated attention from two playful adults. Tony entertained all with his little-boy antics, and eight-year-old Jamie blessed the ladies with her good-natured ways.

Florida law and the responsibilities of parenting Heather sent us once more to unfamiliar territory. A social worker came from the state office to recruit homes for about a dozen especially difficult-to-place children. A pamphlet catalogued the waiting youths, ages ranging from babies to teens, or sibling groups. Some had photographs, some didn't. They had physical or developmental problems, or were black, biracial, or older than seven. Much information hadn't been updated in five years. Poor Heather—her blurb might have said, "Thought to be deaf, blind, and retarded;

unable to sit, eat, or breathe on her own." None of it held true any longer.

One specific child was featured with a poster-sized portrait. She explained, "the troubled ten-year-old girl needs an adoptive family in which she can learn trust. She can't live with young children; she'd harm them," the woman said, without batting an eye. "Remember, your first obligation is to your existing family. A man with whom I placed a troubled child divorced both his first and second wives and refuses to recognize the destructiveness of the adopted daughter," she said.

"When the adoption works and you rekindle a child's spirit, the joy is indescribable. You're taking a risk, a calculated risk. If it becomes a certain risk, bail out. Should it come to that, no one will understand the magnitude of your loss. No one will send sympathy cards."

Continuing in the same vein, the second session was more depressing. All attendees tenaciously hung on. "Most placements have good endings, but tough beginnings are normal. Oftentimes a child may act out in a sexual manner. Any idea how you might prepare your family ahead of time?" she asked.

"Define to a child what is appropriate and what is not," recommended one classmate.

"Read books about abuse to your sons and daughters. Hopefully they'll confide if anything funny happens," a shy lady said.

"Don't assume a child will confide if he is mistreated, just because you've discussed the issue," someone else warned. "It's too perilous. Abusers, even teenage ones, are sneaky, maybe threatening. The situation is bewildering, especially if the perpetrator is someone the child trusts."

Medically needy kids seemed simpler to Jim and me. Physical illness we understood, yet Alex's rejection was troubling. If Heather died, how would Jamie and Tony react? Could her tenuous hold on life harm their developing psyches? If the unspeakable happened and Heather passed on, we'd feel privileged to have shared a little of life with her, wouldn't we?

A soft-spoken woman walked with me around the corner to the coffee pot. "If you have a minute, I've got to get something off my chest," she said. "They gloss over reality with innocent-sounding words, but don't mention the thing that happened to my friend's little daughter—full-blown rape by the adopted son without any forewarning." Her voice quavered. "The worst part is the boy admitted his guilt. HRS counselors couldn't accept it and accused my friends of mistreatment and tried to invent a reason to take their biological children into custody." She stopped to regain her composure.

"The system's all wrong! In their zeal to prosecute, they made up allegations, like saying a supermarket cashier would testify that they bought nothing but peanut butter to feed their kids. Pure poppycock." She stamped her foot. "Authorities couldn't accept that guidance and love aren't always enough. Psychological damage can run too deep."

"Keep good records." It was the second time someone gave me that warning. "Less proof is needed to take a child from his parents than to convict someone of a crime. Only a preponderance of evidence is required, not clear and convincing facts. Anonymous gossip can stand as solid testimony, without any verification as to its validity. Don't misunderstand me," she emphasized. "We've adopted two abused youngsters, and they are heaven's gifts."

"That ostracized girl on the poster," I ventured. "Even if an adopting family doesn't have children, what about the neighbors' youngsters?"

"It is a problem," she said, "but things aren't always how they are presented. A good child may be bad, or a supposedly bad child may be good. Reliable investigations take time. Overworked caseworkers sometimes slant the story or make up big fat lies to justify erroneously removing a child and ignore tons of evidence that show it was a mistake. Poverty-stricken parents have no money to hire an attorney to express their side of the story or to file a lawsuit."

She told how her adopted sons remembered hiding in a bathroom with their mom and grandma. Police battered down the door and dragged the boys away. She had a chance to review their file. A supposed cigarette burn on one boy's arm. Who did it? the parent? a teacher? Accidental? Records said the father inflicted it on purpose to force the mother to retract testimony concerning insurance fraud that benefitted his relative. The boys were never returned to their mother's care. HRS jostled them through thirty different foster homes before they became members of the soft-spoken woman's family. She stopped talking, closed her eyes. Deep furrows lined her brow.

CHAPTER 15]
ANOTHER WAY

An invisible line distinguished us from the rest of the drab, wide-open hospital lobby. I was sitting in the waiting-for-your-child-in-surgery nook pretending to read, biding the surreal, drawn-out passing of time. The month between tracheal dilations had again hurtled by. A volunteer snapped his fingers to gain my attention. "Someone from the O.R. wants to speak with you."

He motioned for me to follow along through several corridors. I did not allow any theories to enter my mind as to the reason for his request, or I might have collapsed. In the operating room suites he introduced me to a young nurse clad in the usual blue scrubs and surgical protective garb that left only her eyes visible. White paper surgical booties covered her shoes. A flimsy cap resembling one for the shower covered her hair. She slipped her face mask down below her chin. Her lips began moving.

She reassured me that surgery went safely, then helped clad me in surgical attire similar to hers, and walked me to the immediate post-operative recovery area. "We can't calm her," she disclosed. "That's why I sent for you. Your little girl is sobbing uncontrollably. Her trach keeps plugging. Though it is against the rules, would you please come mollify her?" she begged.

Heather gurgled blood-tinged mucous bubbling up from tissue traumatized by the dilating rods. I suctioned using our parent-devised gentler technique. I soothed her. After a few hours, the mucilaginous rivulet abated.

In preparation for moving her to the pediatric floor, the pleasant nurse changed the lighted oxygen-level sensor pad on Heather's finger to one that was battery powered. To ensure her safe transfer, a portable alarm tracked her heart rate as I kept hold of her hand and walked alongside the rolling crib, happy that our destination was the monitored ward on the regular pediatric floor, not the PICU.

"Are these arrangements better?" the surgeon asked when he stopped in.

"Terrific, thanks for facilitating it." Each parent was allotted a cot to stretch out on, and could sleep if tired. Quarters were tight yet wonderfully accommodating. One parent was permitted to stay continuously day and night.

The surgeon believed he'd opened up the glistening scar in Heather's airway enough for success. "Wait two days for the swelling to decrease; then place the Passy-Muir® speaking valve over the trach tube opening," he said.

Bob, the bearded nurse, reviewed what we already knew. "A one-way flap opens with each inhalation but closes on exhalation, forcing air out through her vocal cords and nose or mouth, creating a beautiful potential for spoken words. Or tragedy!" He drilled into us the dire consequence of asphyxiation. A safety feature was built into the design, but wasn't guaranteed. If scar tissue remained or re-expanded and obstructed her trachea, any exhaled breaths were blocked from escaping through her nose or mouth or out of the closed one-way flap.

If such a scenario occurred, her lungs would remain overfilled with air, yet need oxygen. Air hunger would drive desperate attempts at tiny inhalations, destined to fail as there would be no more space for breath in the lungs. Mounting pressures of excess volumes of air trapped in her lungs theoretically would explosively pop off the entire speaking valve device, allowing normal trach breathing to resume. "But the safety feature doesn't always work. Keep Heather and her breathing under constant surveillance whenever she wears the valve."

The charming possibility that Heather's spoken words might soon lace the air enchanted our imagination. To hear her sing, to hear her laugh . . . would her melodies be whispery or bold, squeaky or exuberant, dainty or bear a Southern twang? Or defeat, what if there was no voice? Mixed emotions tiptoed into the dream. What if the stupendous possibility for voice was permanently snatched away?

For three days after the dilation, the dream subsisted as fact. Stalling. Fidgeting. Then came the moment, Jim boldly fitted the magical speaking valve onto Heather's trach. In great expectation, my hand lingered close to feel that first warm, humid, beautiful breath streaming out of her nose. No draft. Jim grabbed a Kleenex. He held the tissue near her nostrils. No flutter. She tugged in tiny trach breaths and her abdominal muscles contracted. The valve's thin, translucent exit flap bulged yet kept resolutely shut. Heather's lip quivered, and her color began to fade. The safety feature bombed. No popping-off of the speaking valve happened.

"This is crazy," Jim hissed and plucked off the offending device. The doctor had admonished us not to quit too soon. We experimented twice more to no avail. Clearly scar tissue still clogged her airway.

What if she never becomes able to talk? She'd grow frustrated if only her family understood her signed language. Maybe the deaf community would embrace her. Heather'd be more content in a social group where she could converse, wouldn't she? Combined abilities to sign and hear might be an asset, or make her so different that the deaf would reject her? Maybe after the next bronch, maybe then she'd have a voice. . . .

At the city pool three mornings a week, Jamie sprang off a diving block and swam laps with fifty other young athletes. While she improved the form of her arms knifing through the water and the power of her kicks, Tony and Heather scampered over to the swings at the nearby play area. Big brother took charge of teaching little sister the to-and-fro leg pumping action.

We walked back over to the pool toward the end of swim practice. The young competitors sprinted in practice relay races and individual events. "Go Jamie! Pass that girl, go, go, go! Faster!" Tony chanted. Jamie surged ahead. "Jamie won!" he exclaimed. He danced a little victory jig.

"Jamie's swimming," I signed.

"Me swimming," Heather signed in response.

"You can't," I signed and pointed to her trach, trying to explain how water would flood into her lungs. Jim and I so hoped that one day her airway would be healed and that she could swim. We longed to show her the underwater splendor of Florida's coral reefs.

A mother pushing her infant in a stroller stopped to ask me a question. Heather squatted down and scrutinized the three-month-old.

"Baby," I signed.

"Baby," Heather signed and moved to touch the infant, her fingers accidentally brushing an eyelid before gently lighting on his head.

"Whoops, sorry," I said. "Sometimes she's a trifle clumsy." The woman stole a glance at the trach jutting from Heather's neck. She seemed about to say something, but faltered.

"A surgeon is fixing her airway; one day she'll talk," I assured her, addressing her unspoken misgivings, thus gaining a new friend who enjoyed sharing the vision. Mentioning that Heather might never speak caused people to subtly distance themselves.

Afterward we followed a path to a bricked square where the pigeons roosted. We'd brought a loaf of stale bread. Heather pulled off small crumbs and dropped them at her feet. She stayed as still as a statue and soon had cooing, slate-colored birds strutting across her shoes. Tony attempted the same. Impatience won, and his boisterous movements set them all to flight.

July 20 rolled around, and Heather's two-year birthday. We heralded the event with a family picnic at one of Florida's largest sinkholes. Tall spruce and longleaf pines ring the top. Down below is a shimmering pond. Devil's Millhopper—its name derives from a folklore explanation of the fossil bones and shells unearthed at the bottom of the deep pit. The story goes that the Devil excavated the earth, shaping the depression into a deep and narrow cone-like funnel, but instead of tossing grain into the hopper, he plunged animals to their death and dragged them down under to populate his fiery abode.

Perched on a viewing platform, we gazed at the steeply descending slopes covered with lush resurrection ferns and patches of moss. Cool moisture flowed up from the depths. Heather motioned to Jim and climbed aboard his back to catch a piggyback ride. He carried her down the 236 spiraling steps, descending through verdant foliage and ending in a boardwalk that encircles the spring water pool. I toted her emergency kit loaded with suction machine, nebulizer, spare trach, and resuscitative ambu bag. It still followed her everywhere like a shadow. Jamie carted the snacks.

Marveling at the richness of our family, Jim and I relaxed. All five of us frittered away the afternoon searching out frogs and turtles and crawly things. Heather dashed around the planking with her siblings. Tony tossed rocks into the pond. A great blue heron flew overhead and landed on its large stick nest to feed its squawking young.

Time to leave, Jim lowered himself into a squat. "Departure, hop on up," he said, inviting Heather to climb aboard.

Heather shook her head 'no,' and resolutely refused the ride. She patted her open palm on her chest, "Me," she signed. Jim attempted to dissuade her, but she again signed the word for "me," insisting *me do it*. With determination, she ascended one step after another until she'd climbed up all 236 steps. Proud confidence shined on her face as she trotted the last half-mile of trail to the parking lot. No shortness of breath. No emergency breathing treatments. The health of her lungs had improved so much. Maybe she could get the trach out. Hope welled up like the waters below.

Incredulous I know, that she climbed all those steps, but she did. A feat that very few two-years-old would even want to achieve, but Heather possessed an understated pleasant stubbornness to exist when necessary as a cocoon, but when possible to achieve the potential of unique Heather.

Back home, neighbors joined us for birthday cake. Jim lifted her into the high chair. A rainbow-colored party hat rested on her head, with hair bangs peeking under. Her two top and bottom teeth had finally erupted, and her weight had crept above the twenty-pound mark. She got us all laughing by making silly monster faces that she'd learned from Tony.

Jamie adorned radiant Heather with gifts of gaudy beads, bracelets, and long dangling earrings. Bejeweled Heather lifted her arms and hugged her sister and bestowed a gentle kiss, the *first time* ever. Heavens waltzed in celebration. At last the child could display the love that multiplied in her soul.

Jim lit the two candles, and we sang a rousing chorus of "Happy Birthday." He positioned a loose-fitting plastic mask over the trach tube to prevent crumbs of chocolate cake from landing in it. Feeding herself like a big girl, Heather spooned in cake and ice cream, letting melting sweetness run out the corners of her mouth.

As a precaution, we bathed her in the kitchen sink instead of the tub to avoid chances of her slipping under the water. She still had the gastrostomy feeding button in her abdomen. Marveling at her, I pondered the earlier predictions that she was deaf, blind, and retarded. What tragedies befall children whose parents accept such limitations as fact?

Mom again pressed me to tend to one of her big concerns. Heather tilted her head sideways when she walked. Her eyes sometimes wandered independent of each other. I'd noticed but shoved the observation aside, perhaps fearing a need for additional surgery.

The pediatrician confirmed that my mom was correct to be worried. Misaligned eyes create double-vision. "Her brain will shut off nerve impulses to one eye, effectively blinding it, to

eliminate the blurred images if not corrected," he said. His staff scheduled an appointment with the ophthalmologist for the next day.

That doctor gave good news after his examination. "Wearing glasses will correct her focus and align her eyes. Her eye muscles are balanced. No surgery is necessary."

Heather looked cute wearing pink frames that looped over and behind the top of her ears to keep them secured. Showing off her new eyeglasses, she bobbed about while wearing her favorite tasseled yellow knitted hat and the necklace of colorful jangling fruit.

Becoming somewhat cynical: did the therapies benefit Heather or the learning students or someone's paycheck? Did anyone stop to think it through? Could we refuse as we were only foster parents? Also feeling impatient, when might we start our adoption classes?

Boredom, hunger, and fatigue pestered Heather and me. Monthly bronchoscopy had come around again too soon. Waiting in our corner of the main lobby, surrounded by multitudes of people grew tedious. Four hours had passed since first being notified of an indefinite delay. There wasn't a pediatric space available in the surgical recovery room. "Home is fifteen minutes away. Maybe we can leave and come back when surgery is ready?" I asked. The clerk refused.

Heather had not drank any fluids or eaten any nourishment since the night before. Eating before surgery was prohibited. Sojourning in the cafeteria wasn't possible for that and an additional reason. In those days thick clouds of cigarette smoke hung heavy and masked any aromas from the kitchen. Not good for her breathing or mine.

Midafternoon a surgical nurse came for her. To bide my time while the surgeon dilated her scarred airway, I began my fake book-reading. *Déjà vu.* Fake reading interrupted by what was becoming a familiar request from the recovery room. "There is no quieting your daughter." As I followed along, I asked the nurse about Alexander, the small boy with a trach whose adoptive parents had returned him.

"Alex still lives in PICU. Almost three years old, he's never left except for those couple of weeks. With frequent exposure to illness, he stays sickly," she replied. A tragedy, we both agreed.

Rounding the corner was my Heather. All I saw was flailing limbs, a contorting face, and inaudible sobs. Under the crib rail, I felt for and released the lowering latch. Crying Heather scrambled to me. Copious gurgles sprayed from her trach, splattering her neck and gown and my blouse. I wiped away the mess with delicate strokes and consoled her as she scrunched closer.

Once the nurse was sure Heather was stable, she transferred Heather in the rolling crib to the pediatric ward as I tagged along. I was surprised to find young Samantha and her mom resting in the adjacent bed.

"You always seem so relaxed," Samantha's mom commented.

"It's different for Jim and me," I admitted. "We chose Heather and her problems. No mourning the loss of idealistic notions about the fun of raising a healthy child, when instead a new baby is born gravely ill, and serious forever changes follow."

Jim took over tending Heather when he got off work. It was August 2 and happened to be Jamie's ninth birthday. Jim's parents drove up from Miami for the occasion. Minus Jim, we celebrated at the Melting Pot, a local fondue restaurant. Afterward, I traded with Jim and slept at the hospital.

When the surgeon came by on morning rounds, I explained about the speaking valve and very scary because the safety pop-it-off failed. He didn't say much in reply. I briefed him that the adoption was almost finalized. "Would you fill out the required report of her medical history?" I asked.

"Can't do it; I'm too busy," he snapped and walked out.

Aghast at his callous brush-off—no minutes to fill out a few forms so an abandoned child can have a permanent family? No, you won't be operating on my little girl anymore, not once I have a choice. Was he more receptive to parents who could opt to seek medical care for their children elsewhere? Few doctors accepted government-sponsored Medicaid. Reimbursement often didn't cover the overhead expense of treating the patient; instead it created a financial loss.

Computers were not yet widely available. That evening after bringing Heather home, I left her with Jim and headed to the medical library. Maybe there was a newer treatment. I scanned the titles of rows of reference books. I searched the medical terms *subglottic stenosis* (tracheal scarring) and *bronchopulmonary dysplasia*

(diseased lungs). Around me I piled up volumes that listed indexes and abstracts of relevant articles. I sat on the floor and read.

Periodically, the whine of a copying machine interrupted the quiet, as did the sounds of a librarian punching a stapler, crumpling paper, and opening a squeaky drawer. After turning hundreds of pages and finding nothing, I walked over to where I could phone my brother. Mark had an idea. At Vanderbilt University he had access to a computerized Medline search, and he volunteered to run one.

The promised list arrived by mail in a couple of days. I tore open the envelope and read through all the abstracts. Jim rushed to the medical library and copied the full article of any that were promising. More valuable than gold, the grit of the material revealed that monthly dilations were considered obsolete and thought to increase scarring. Dilating efforts might be effective in a few select cases.

"Hey, Jim!" I called out when my perusal yielded more treasure. "A Dr. Cotton in Cincinnati has invented a groundbreaking procedure. He harvests a sliver of rib cartilage, then grafts it into the scarred trachea to enlarge it. It's called a laryngotracheoplasty."

"Sounds intriguing, but don't get too optimistic," he cautioned. "Out-of-state Medicaid poses an insurance problem, and who knows whether the operation can benefit Heather?"

"But maybe it will."

"And maybe it won't," he answered.

"Then the solution will be that there is none. Nothing, no solution at all," I said. "And we'll enjoy each day as it unfolds." An ideal easier achieved in theory, than in reality, I admitted.

One of Heather's HRS social workers verified that seeking a second medical opinion, even in another state, was permissible.

"Sounds like providence. Jump on it," she encouraged. "We like parents to be aggressive advocates."

"Terrific," I replied. "I already called Ohio and left a message with the surgeon's assistant."

CHAPTER 16]
MOVING ON

That night Jim fired up the grill. Sitting around the dining table, we were stringing vegetables on kabob sticks when Dr. Cotton's secretary called with information. So fast, the secretary could have scheduled Heather an expedited appointment if the adoption was final. Our private health insurance plan would have covered the examination and any necessary surgery in Ohio. As it stood, we'd have to secure Florida Medicaid's written approval for treatment and their commitment to pay the bill in full.

Jim rubbed his chin, and that little muscle near his ear twitched. "We'll obtain approval," he said, and he was thinking at super speed, out-pacing me. "Maybe a temporary move to Cincinnati would be wise in case she has complications, but what about employment?"

"If I'm not choosy, I can get hired as a nurse pronto. Perhaps your boss would grant you a leave of absence. While we're in Ohio, you could take the easy job," I said, being sarcastic, "be the stay-at-home dad and take care of the kids."

Before that scenario went any further, my brother suggested a prospect closer to home. "Hold on," he said. "Dr. Jay Werkhaven just came on staff here. He knows a children's ear, nose, and throat surgeon in Jacksonville—Dr. Bruce Maddern. They studied together at the Children's Hospital of Pittsburgh under the tutelage of Drs. Charles Bluestone and Sylvan Stool, two of the founders of the new field."

Pediatric otolaryngologists complete an additional two-year fellowship after the initial five-year ENT surgical residency. At the time, there were only about fifty in the whole world. Dr. Cotton was also one of them.

"Call Nemours Children's Clinic, and if a physician's referral is required, give Werkhaven's name. Once you meet Dr. Maddern," my brother insisted, "follow your original plans to move nearer to Mom and Dad, instead of to Cincinnati. Tell Jim not to worry, a medic helicopter could transport her to Jacksonville in thirty minutes if something emergent went wrong."

How stupendous if Dr. Maddern really was the "Voice Giver"? If he could get the trach out and she could talk? Not only talk, but without a trach, Heather could safely play in a sandbox or eat drippy, flavored, shaved ice, and go to friends' sleepovers. Swimming and snorkeling among the brilliant coral reefs would become a reality. Sometimes the ability to swim without drowning seemed almost as important as uttering spoken words.

Shifting from my dreamy musings, I asked the question that would surely blow it out of the water: "Does Dr. Maddern accept Medicaid?"

"I don't know, but if he likes treating children with complicated airway and hearing disorders, he'd have to," my brother Mark asserted.

Dr. Bruce Maddern's new office was open and ready for business. His receptionist confirmed his acceptance of Medicaid. She scheduled Heather's appointment for the first week in September. If Florida had cherry blossoms, they would have burst into bloom at those words.

Crossing off the days, we'd reached the Monday that Jim had circled in red on the calendar. Having successfully navigated six months of not feeding her through the button in her abdomen, its removal was scheduled for her next clinic appointment.

I didn't bother asking the surgeon a second time about the needed papers. The pulmonary nurse specialist filled out the formal health history. She had one of the lung doctors review and sign it. If the adoption could be finalized, we'd have more options for healing Heather, and perhaps more financial responsibility. The HRS social worker explained, "after the adoption is finalized, the state pays any expenses stemming from documented existing or previous medical conditions. Unrelated or undocumented illness will come out of your pocket." Supposedly foster children who become adopted kept Medicaid until age eighteen. No one pointed out the fine print: the state could negate the agreement at any time.

At the clinic appointment, Heather sat in my lap, while Tony held her hand. I lifted up her polka-dotted sun dress and opened the air-mattress like plug of the feeding button. Inside of her stomach, a soft, mushroom-shaped anchor kept the device in place. A doctor-in-training threaded a metal probe through the center hole to straighten the soft anchor into a slender pencil-shape.

Gently he tugged out the device, followed by leaking, clumpy stomach juices. Heather and Tony wrinkled their noses, but no drama. Both were accustomed to medical procedures. To obstruct the leaking tract, the doctor inserted an adult-sized urinary catheter. He inflated its balloon inside her stomach to tether it there.

"As her body forms scar tissue to fill the tract, replace the catheter with one that is narrower." The doctor handed me an assortment of smaller sizes. "Repeat the process until a minuscule hole remains, then remove the catheter and leave it out. Cover with a bandage until it fully heals and seals off."

At her follow-up Gainesville clinic appointment I lifted the lower edge of Heather's shirt to show her 'ouchie' to the doctor-in-training. I told him about all the on-going problems, despite our following his instructions.

With awkward and annoying messiness, Heather's gastrostomy hole stubbornly remained open and refused to heal. Despite smearing the area with ointment and padding it with gauze, stomach acids dribbled out around the catheter and ate away the tender skin of her tummy. Sometimes the excess length of catheter, which we hid in a neat loop, uncoiled and snaked out under her clothing in full view of strangers. Even worse, the balloon anchor kept popping. The whole apparatus would fall out in public places, and streams of semidigested ooze leaked everywhere.

The doctor conferred with his attending physician. Surgical closure of the gastrostomy hole was slated for October 23 in Gainesville. Jim circled the date on the calendar.

The day of the pivotal take-a-chance and seek a second opinion in Jacksonville arrived.

"Morning, Sunshine," Jim said when waking Heather before daybreak. The early rising stirred some apprehension into her. She signed the telling question by make-believe spooning food toward her mouth and looking inquisitively for an answer. "Yes, you can eat. No surgery today, only a doctor's appointment."

Eggs sizzled in peppered butter. Jim sprinkled cheddar cheese on top. Once melted, he flipped them onto plates and spread strawberry jam onto the toast. We ate our fill.

"Breakfast was delicious; thanks so very much."

"Drive safely, Fan," Jim said, addressing me by an affectionate nickname, and he bade us good luck. Heather seemed contented in her car seat with the distractions of gazing out the window and her brother's chatty silliness. Throughout the two-hour drive to

Jacksonville, hopefulness propagated imaginings of increasingly wondrous possibilities.

Road construction didn't slow midmorning traffic as we entered the city. Skyscrapers populated the river banks. As the exit to Prudential Drive loomed, I put on my blinker; but cars blocked my way to changing lanes, and we zipped over the flowing St. Johns River via the Main Street Bridge. Attractive steel girders painted blue formed an intricate lattice-like tunnel framed by sturdy towers that periodically lifted the entire center section to allow cruising cargo ships to pass through.

After a few course corrections, I veered off onto calmer streets. Railroad crossbars lowered at the second intersection. Warning lights flashed as an approaching freight train chugged onward. Infinitely long, Tony counted each railway car. I could see our destination—the tall medical office building that interconnected with Wolfson Children's Hospital and Baptist Medical Center.

After maneuvering the van into a tight parking spot, I brushed cookie crumbs off Tony and Heather, mopped their faces with a damp cloth, and changed them into fresh clothes. We headed for the lobby. Tony pressed the elevator button, and we were transported up to the destination office. A few other children waited at a cute kid-sized table.

Dr. Maddern's practice was part of the multispecialty Nemours Children's Clinic. Tony picked up a coloring book: "Pine Trees, Railroads, and Kids." The title is one of the clinic's slogans and reflects the foundation's origin and generous goals. He turned the pages while I read.

In 1935 a bequest from Alfred I. duPont established Nemours. DuPont's friend, Edward Ball, helped with its expansion. Both of their companies (St. Joe Paper Company and Florida East Coast Railway) donated substantial amounts of money. Part of Nemours' impressive mission is "to provide leadership, institutions, and services to restore and improve the health care of children through treatment and programs not readily available, with one high standard of quality and distinction regardless of the recipient's financial status." My optimism continued to increase.

Sherri, the office nurse, showed us to an exam room. She asked questions about Heather's health and jotted down the answers. When finished she stuck the new chart into a plastic holder that was mounted in the hallway. Restless from the drive and now in privacy, Tony and Heather raced around the room. When they heard a quiet knock they plopped into chairs and sat without wiggling.

In walked Dr. Maddern, he shook my hand warmly and immediately bent his knees and crouched down to chat with Heather at her level, his moustache easing upward in a smile. Heather touched his nametag then rested her hand on top of his wrist. All the while he observed her breathing. I sensed competence as he explained options, using an anatomical model to add clarity.

"I'll do a diagnostic laryngoscopy and bronchoscopy to thoroughly examine her larynx and airways. There won't be any attempts at dilation. First, she'll be under light sedation, so her vocal cords will still move, and I can observe them; then heavier anesthesia. Laser surgery is often sufficient for children like Heather. The beam can evaporate scar tissue." He explained how the laser can focus on a spot as small as a pinpoint. Its concentrated beam of light destroys the targeted cells while those nearby remain unharmed.

"If the scarring is severe, she'll need airway reconstruction, probably the LTP (laryngotracheoplasty) that you read about. The beauty of the LTP procedure is that the cartilaginous graft will grow with her. Afterward, she's unlikely to require more surgery." He explained how he cuts out a small section of her rib cartilage and sculpts it into a diamond shape. The scarred trachea is incised vertically, and the edges pulled open to accommodate the graft, which is sutured into place, enlarging and creating an open tubular airway. He smiled, and his eyes sparkled with confidence that comes from experience.

"Here is a prescription for a pre-operative EKG (electrocardiogram) and pulmonary function studies," he said. "The tests serve as yardsticks to determine if she can handle an increase in the work of breathing. Nose breathing takes three times as much effort as inhaling and exhaling through a trach."

"Her lungs have strengthened," I said. "Something amazing happened on her birthday. She climbed up the 236 steps at Devil's Millhopper, all by herself. Never short of breath, never got winded."

"That sounds promising," he said, shifting his attention to Heather, showing her a cheerful face, then became serious. "One obstacle, Heather is technically a foster child. For any surgical procedures that are done under anesthesia, a judge has to issue a court order allowing the team to proceed. We know how to get one; we've done it before."

"Maybe we can sidestep the issue and get the adoption finalized. The last hurdle is HRS placing a classified ad for an unknown father to come forward. The notice runs for several weeks," I said.

"Can you obtain copies of her previous surgical and X-ray reports, so I can review them?" he asked.

"Sure, the parcel of medical papers might measure a few inches thick." I moved my thumb and index finger apart, gauging my estimate. I promised to mail them within the week.

"Any more questions?" he asked.

"Does hospital policy permit Jim or me to stay with her, even overnight? Are there different restrictions for parents visiting in the PICU than on the pediatric floor?

"Wolfson Children's Hospital almost mandates that parents stay around the clock to care for their child," he answered.

Nurse Sherri peeked in. "All arranged. Heather is set on the surgical calendar for the tenth of October." It seemed a dream. In a month, Maddern would determine the best approach to fixing Heather's airway. If lasering alone could eliminate her airway scarring, maybe just maybe, Heather would get the trach out not too long after.

"Thanks," I said. The word felt inadequate.

Arriving home, I told Jim all about it, then called my siblings, and Mom and Dad. After relaying the details of the intriguing appointment to my sister, she pestered Jim and me to commit to moving back home.

"Maybe it is possible," I replied. "If travelling to Jacksonville for Heather's medical care, we could as easily commute from Cocoa Beach."

"Cocoa Beach is terrific," she said, "ocean swimming, boating on the river, and time with Mom and Dad." She'd relocated there from Memphis with her husband and two young sons. They'd purchased an older home a half-mile from our parents.

Out front one of the impromptu street gatherings was assembling. Tony joined his buddies, Tom and Ross. They clambered onto their trikes and peeled out like race drivers. Heather followed along on her own ride—a sit-on and scoot-along inchworm on wheels. Her exuberance was wordless and silent, while the boys' expressions were chatty and boisterous.

Jim mentioned our tentative moving plans to a neighbor who lived on the corner. "A lady at work expressed an interest in buying a house in Valwood; I'll mention yours," he offered. Three days later his nurse co-worker stopped by to look around our home. A kind woman, Anita got to talking and shared an adoption story of her own, personal and tragic.

Her best friend died, leaving behind a husband and young daughter. The grieving widower asked Anita to raise the child because prior to that blow, he already suffered from a major psychiatric illness. The father trusted Anita and knew she'd keep him an integral part of his daughter's life.

"After three years of his illness persisting without remission, he asked me to formally adopt his daughter. We researched the law," Anita said. "To accomplish that, he had to voluntarily relinquish his parental rights. We dodged the one other possible hitch. In Texas at that time, HRS only allowed married couples to adopt. No problem, we thought. I was engaged, and 'everyone would live happily ever after'," she said long-suffering, pausing to maintain composure.

"By terrible fate; my fiancé died in an automobile crash. On that technicality, HRS ripped away my little girl and gave her to strangers for permanent adoption. It felt like a kidnapping. Poor child lost her biological mother, then me—her second mother, and her dad, all of us forever." I listened. How does one recover from all that? I hoped I'd never have to be that stoic.

As for purchasing our home, Anita brought over a written offer later that week. Jim harbored a few reservations about uprooting the family, so he countered with a higher selling price. Anita agreed and wrote out a deposit check.

Life tumbled forward with a continuing abundance of unanticipated ventures. The search began for a home near to Cocoa Beach. Simultaneously Jim and I contemplated prospects for work and debated when to give notice to our employment managers.

CHAPTER 17] NEW DIRECTIONS

Steep prices vanquished any ideas of purchasing an abode in mint condition. With Jim's blessings, Jamie, Tony, and I travelled to my parents for a weekend of house hunting. He stayed behind with Heather. That way we avoided the packing and unpacking of all her equipment.

Mom and I scanned the newspaper and found an ad for an open house at a handyman's special. "Don't stop!" Jamie beseeched me, when she saw the overgrown mess. Three large stumps rose above an unkempt overgrown lawn that could have served as a prop for a horror movie. On the compelling side, the house sat on a double lot with mature oak trees. Both features were uncommon so near the beach. Despite Jamie's protests, I parked and got out of the car. Then, I waylaid a man strolling down the street.

"Excuse me, how much is this house worth?" I asked.

"Maybe seventy thousand. It's in bad shape and has stood empty for longer than a year," he said. "Renters abused it. We watched them get raided by the police on a few occasions. A young family taking over the place would be nice."

Holes where fists had punched through doors and walls illustrated how greatly the former tenants differed from the neighbors, serene retirees who'd moved in when their children were

141

young. Water stains mapped out plumbing leaks. Animal hair matted the carpet. The house was almost thirty years old, so it had weathered any tropical storm or hurricane that had blown through. I explored nearby streets. The kids could bike to school. The ocean was only a half-mile to the east, and the river was three houses to the west.

My parents drove down and met me there. Dad and I crawled through the attic, probing for termites. Mom yanked up a corner of the filthy carpet. "There's terrazzo under here. Polish it up, and that faux marble will shine," she said. Water and electricity were shut down. No way to test the working condition of many things. I worried that major appliances might be broken.

"Renters lived here, didn't they?" Dad asked. "I bet the AC, oven, and plumbing work," he speculated. "Basic structure is solid. Buy it at a bargain price, then it won't matter what requires fixing or replacing."

Mom figured an offer to purchase it as-is would be snatched up. "Decline any additional inspections. Strike out such clauses in the typed offer, and any other deal-breakers or those that cost the seller repair money. Give him only five days to accept or reject," Mom insisted, and added more emphatic. "Heather's surgery is fast approaching."

I phoned Jim and bubbled enthusiasm about the location as if I'd won a lottery. I'd overheard another prospective buyer's bid. "Since your folks agree, go ahead and make the offer. Top the other offer by five thousand." he suggested, equally intrigued.

"Cross your fingers," I said.

The realtor, who had waited patiently as we rummaged the house, formalized the written offer and promised to soon be in touch.

Dad suggested a refreshing walk on the beach. Jamie and Tony waded in the surf and poked about, collecting a few seashells.

Farther along on the other side of the sand dunes and boardwalk, we crossed the beach access road to Wendy's. Hungry, we ordered cheeseburgers and french fries and sipped cold chocolate shakes. Reluctant to leave, we hugged my parents good-bye, and I drove the kids back to Gainesville.

Life accelerated into the super-fast lane. Honoring the time window, the seller signed the deal! Finding new employment moved up to the top of our to-do list. At a hospital near to the fixer-upper, I spoke with the nurse-manager of the labor-and-delivery unit. "I have a lot of experience. I bought a house and need a job," I told her that bluntly.

At the in-person interview I explained about our child-care dilemma. Comprehending the complexity of Heather's health issues, the nurse manager agreed to schedule me to work only evening or weekend shifts. Mandatory hospital-wide orientation, for the first week would be day shift, Monday through Friday. Jim would care for Heather, I assured her. She hired me.

Blessings come, sometimes disguised as an unsettling call from a surgical nurse.

"Dr. Martin scratched your daughter's gastrostomy closure that is scheduled for October 23rd," she said.

"Okay, on what day is it rescheduled?" I asked.

"It isn't," she said. "He won't perform the operation."

"Then which other doctor is surgically closing the leaking hole in her belly?" I asked.

"No physician here will do it," the nurse said.

"Why?" I asked, dumbfounded.

"The doctor didn't provide a reason," she said. Her resolute voice ended the conversation.

Hmmm, a really wanting to throw a tantrum crossed my mind, but instead I quietly asked my husband, "What now?"

"Either the surgeon didn't believe Heather eats, or he'd refused because of our cancelling all of Heather's upcoming bronchoscopies and tracheal dilations," Jim replied. Followed by a quick thinking, "maybe call Jacksonville?"

Nurse Sherri listened, and spoke in soft, calming voice. "Maybe a Nemours surgeon can close the hole in her abdomen. Don't fret if it takes a few days to get an answer." It took less than one hour. "Dr. Webb says okay, but she must come to his office prior to surgery day. How about Tuesday?"

"Sure," I answered.

"This way is better—one less episode of Heather having to undergo anesthesia. Dr. Maddern will perform the diagnostic airway procedure, and then to follow, Dr. Webb will surgically close the gastrostomy hole. All procedures will occur in the same operating room," Sherri said.

"We really appreciate your assistance," I said.

Auspiciously, a gift dropped from heaven on October 2, one year from that night I woke Jim, and he thought I had lost my mind. One year from when I had first uttered the strangest of words, "there's a little girl . . . we should adopt her." Without fanfare, inside a plain envelope, in the routinely delivered mail, the declaration arrived—legal, stamped adoption papers. Heather Elizabeth Giganti was truly ours!

The birth certificate listed us, James Gregory and Ann Widick Giganti, as Heather's parents from the moment she was born. Period. Nothing referred to an adoption or pointed to her original birth name. Jim and I could sign medical papers and surgical permissions without any limitations. Court orders wouldn't be necessary. Thank goodness.

Martha Lott finalized the last required legal details. Jim and I were forever legally Heather's parents, the greatest of understated glories. Mark Hoffenberg created an elegant adoption announcement with his hand-scripted calligraphy. We mailed them out, announcing our joy.

Announcing the adoption
of
Heather Elizabeth Giganti
Born July 20, 1987
Joined our hearts October 3, 1988
Joined our home February 16, 1989
Adopted October 3, 1989
Loved by her family
Ann, Jimmy, Jamie, & Tony

Late morning of October 9th, we'd fueled the car, and all was ready for our drive to Jacksonville. Overnight, we'd bunk at the Pavilion Inn. Convenient, as it connected to the hospital by an enclosed hallway.

We were eager for Dr. Maddern's opinion, but Heather's forehead was too warm, and her trach mucus was an ugly yellow. A respiratory virus had gotten a grip on her. Reluctantly, we cancelled. Dr. Maddern's disappointment hedged through his professionalism. Nurse Sherri reset the procedures for early December.

The finalized sale of our Gainesville home happened too fast. Though it officially belonged to Anita, she graciously let us live there a few extra days, which included Halloween. Chuck and Sherry were hosting the neighborhood's annual haunting extravaganza.

Packing to move occupied Jim and me, while Halloween preparations flavored the day for the children. They crafted a large cardboard box into a ghoulish experience. On each side, they'd colored hoot owls perched on tombstones and floating ghosts haunting an eerie sky. Dare to slip your hand through spider holes, and a child's fingers palpated witches' teeth (candy corn), brittle bones (turkey-legs), and mucky soil filled with worms. Tony mounded red Jell-O over cooked pasta, then submerged his hands in the monster brains and gave chase to his sister. Fleeing Jamie squealed, then pivoted and pelted Tony with two rotting eyes (peeled green grapes).

Haley showed off her beautiful emerald princess gown. Jamie cackled and grabbed her wicked-witch broom. Jessica posed as a mime—face all white and clothes all black.

Dressed only as herself, mute Heather wandered outside over to the birdbath near the front walkway and swirled the water with her fingers. She patted the top of her head, letting rivulets drip down her cheeks. She picked out a decaying leaf and studied it. Jim followed close as Heather crossed the street and meandered through different activities.

A dozen youngsters took turns bobbing for apples. Affable red-haired Sam ducked his head under the water. Tony, Tom, and Ross tossed bean bags at a wooden target. Grown men shot flaming bottle rockets out of soda bottles and tossed lit firecrackers. Jim kept hold of Heather's hand lest she bolt into the exploding fracas in the middle of the road. The ladies chatted about recipes and nothing important. It was too sad to talk about our moving.

Folks on 80th Street always enjoyed each other's friendships, but silent Heather's spiritual draw had united us into an exquisite bouquet. Sherry couldn't stave off tears and stopped her toast, speechless when she presented us with a going-away gift of a cloth-covered album. Talented Mark had photographed family groups.

Farewell notes of various styles, including a poem, were interspersed with the pictures.

For our last busy days, glad tidings and a hot dinner cooked by a neighbor arrived each evening. Mark helped Jim load all of our belongings into a rented U-Haul truck. After stuffing in the last of the chairs, back inside into the living room, we spread sleeping bags out on top of the carpet. Our children plopped down and began calling out silly words to echo in the emptiness of the bare house. Soundless Heather mimicked their body movements, but did not move her lips.

After we locked the house up for our departure, we walked over to Mark and Celeste's home. For the whole year, they'd kept the impending arrival of their newest child low key. While respecting Celeste's desire for privacy, we wanted to see Haley and newborn Nicholas one more time.

Near sunset on November 3 we embarked on the journey south. Halfway there Jim pulled in to one of the turnpike rest stops to buy sodas. Somehow the cool night air shrank the diameter of my fingers, and my wedding band slipped off. After a cursory search and too exhausted to care, I insisted on driving onwards. Jim, equally tired, did not protest.

Due to the shabby condition of the fixer-upper house, the bank refused to lend money or to let us move in, until two pages of mandatory repairs were completed. Fortunately, the contract stipulated that we could store our belongings in the garage.

Mom and Dad invited us to stay with them until all was settled. A little antsy about investing so many dollars and labor before actually owning the house, we nevertheless leapt forward. To knock out the list quickly, Jim and I would have to work together, but how to protect Heather from exposure to air-borne debris and paint fumes?

Fabulous nurse Betsey agreed to care for Heather at my parents' house. She drove down the day after we arrived and stayed for an entire week. Energetic Betsey borrowed a beach bike and toted Heather in its child's seat on excursions to the library and various restaurants for lunch. Mom and Dad offered her a bedroom, but she opted to stay at a friend's oceanside condo.

The extended family pitched in, cleaning dirt-blackened awning windows and fixing their hand-cranks, digging out the sprinkler system, sprigging plugs of grass, patching holes, and applying over thirty gallons of interior paint to faded walls. Professionals replaced the shower-pan liner and rebuilt the interesting square bathtub that was constructed entirely of tile.

Dad was right: the AC cooled, and the oven worked to warm ready-to-eat meals for hungry laborers. Though the original old-style gravel roof kept the house as dry as when it was installed twenty-seven years earlier, the mortgage specialist insisted we update to a shingled roof. When the workers scraped off the old gravel, it rained showers of rubble through the rafters and no-ceiling garage and onto our belongings. Yuck!

We all got emotional when Betsey's stay was up. As a token of our appreciation, we gave her the oversized hammock that she loved to laze in with Heather.

Adopting Heather was like falling into quicksand—unable to move out of the trap without others' help.

Jim and I discussed how much our lifestyle had changed. We'd always prided ourselves on self-reliance. Great numbers of people kept assisting us and an on-going even greater number of new and random acquaintances, collected at our many new stops, some quickly falling off and others sticking for the long haul.

Having a handicapped child instead of a healthy one is like planning a Paris vacation, but instead the airplane lands in Rome. First the vacationers are angry about not touring the Eiffel Tower, viewing a Monet, or floating down the Seine. Acceptance sets in, and they soon discover that Rome has its own wonders, the journey different but fantastic just the same.

Prior to Heather's December 5th appointment in Jacksonville, things were settling into place. Jim landed a job in the administrative computer department at Florida Tech, a local private university. Jamie enrolled in Indialantic Elementary School. We wrapped up the last chunk of home repairs, closed on the house, and moved in. Without true ownership at stake, we'd have dragged it out for decades.

Enjoying our new location, Jim and I woke the kids early to catch a sunrise at the beach. Stopping first at a donut shop, Heather pressed close, both hands on the glass display case and pointed at a glazed cruller. Jamie and Tony each selected a cinnamon twist.

On the wooden deck overlooking the sand dunes, early morning dew dampened the picnic table, but it wasn't too wet to sit down and eat our sweets. In the quiet before dawn, with the sun hidden below the horizon, and while the birds still slept, we scanned the ocean—glassy with tall waves rolling shoreward in clustered sets. After eating the last crumb, Heather burst into a crying fit.

"Sorry, there's no more," I said.

"What's the matter, baby?" Jim asked. Our girl never cried except at the hospital. Jim carried his unhappy daughter down the stairs. On the beach she grew frantic. We became more perplexed.

"It's the roar of the waves crashing on the shore," Jamie proposed. The morning stillness magnified their sounds, and Heather found it terrifying. We left.

On December 5, we arrived at the hospital in Jacksonville and checked in to the Pavilion Inn. Everyone acted so politely and friendly that it seemed we were at Disney World. Heather's time in the operating room was brief. Dr. Maddern sought us out in the comfortable waiting room as soon as he'd finished. "I did some lasering, but the scarring is severe. I couldn't see past her vocal cords; she will need the rib-graft reconstruction." He'd schedule the surgery for the coming spring. "Best to wait until the winter flu season is over," he explained.

Next out to see us was Dr. Webb. All had gone well with closing the leaking tract to her stomach. He recommended a surgeon near our home who could remove the stitches. We cleaned the area twice a day and changed the bandages. Despite meticulous care, the stitched-closed tummy area puffed up, reddened, and inflicted pain. Unfortunately the local surgeon had retired. It was a weekend. No doctor would treat a kid with a trach and an abdominal surgical infection, if he had not performed the surgery. Even worse an out-of-town surgery.

"An abscess is forming. She needs those stitches out," my brother Mark advised. "An emergency room can't turn her away."

Dr. Congenial, the on-call surgeon, came into the cubicle where I waited with Heather in the emergency room. Rude treatment of Medicaid patients, specifically of Heather and myself, was a scenario that I hoped to avoid. Right away I worked "my brother's a surgical resident at Vanderbilt" into the ER conversation. Dr. Congenial gently removed the stitches. Heather didn't flinch or cry.

Two days later at the office follow-up appointment, his partner was on duty. All had been smooth, so I skipped mentioning my brother.

"What antibiotic is she on?" the doctor asked.

"I can't pronounce it, but it's spelled . . ."

"You should have brought the bottle," he snapped. "Don't ever come without it." His disrespectful barrage continued.

"Sorry, I thought the hospital report would detail her medications," I said. Heather crawled into my lap and clung to me.

Dr. Rude continued his tirade while scanning her ER summary. Like a chameleon changes color, the doctor's demeanor flipped, his face broadening from a scowl into a friendly smile. "Oh, you adopted her!" he interjected. For the rest of the appointment his words and actions bubbled with sweetness. He prescribed a different antibiotic and scheduled a follow-up.

I refrained from speaking my mind, but after buckling Heather into the car seat, my suppressed frustration burst loose. I sort of slammed the vehicle's door with braked vigor. "What's the matter with people? A biological mom is dirt, and an adoptive one an angel?" I muttered to the sky. His attitude flipped, but no transformation of my personality, physical self, or financial situation had occurred. I was the same person whom he first despised. All parents who nurture their children are worthy of respect, regardless of their circumstance.

Perhaps it was anxiety about the unfamiliar territory of treating a two-year-old little girl with a trach that triggered Dr. Rude's venom. For the follow-up appointment Jim took Heather. I wouldn't go. Doctor Rude examined her, but came dressed that day in his best behavior. He declared the hole sealed and infection resolved, and then gifted Heather with a little teddy bear.

Soon thereafter a nurse at Children's Medical Services' subjected me to another infuriating lecture about a request for replenishing Heather's medical supplies. "You're way over income. Another child may have to go without. How selfish!"

"I'm a lot of things, but selfish isn't on the inventory," I replied. "We'd end up homeless if we paid for all her supplies. What about our older children? It's not right to jeopardize their future, because we adopted Heather."

"Well, you're not the only family who's ever taken in a child," was her last remark.

More discouragement, at home I opened a letter from the early intervention clinic and read their summary evaluation of Heather, which concluded, "There are no preschools for the severely language impaired."

Bone-tired, my mind, emotions, and body ached as though I'd hand-plowed a field. I leaned my spine against the back porch wall letting gravity ease me down until my behind rested on the polished terrazzo flooring. Its coolness lessened the fatigue in my stretched out bare legs. An evening breeze evaporated the sticky perspiration on my skin. My head drooped until it rested on my shoulder. Cicadas and a deep-throated bullfrog serenaded me.

"Mom, please come play ball with us," Tony urged, Heather one step behind.

"Ask Daddy; Mommy's tired. . . . Jim! Hey Jim!" I called out loudly. "Tony and Heather want to play ball."

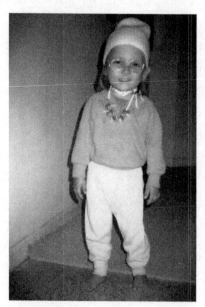

Maybe Heather might talk? Shortly before surgery.

CHAPTER 18]
RAINBOW'S END

Jim and I successfully fumbled through one year of keeping Heather alive. The day of celebration began with goofing off in Florida's pleasant weather. Tiny blossoms covered the tangerine tree in our backyard. For closer inspection of the fragrant flowers, Heather picked a few. "Mama," Heather signed, touching the thumb of her open-hand to her chin, and pointed to a minuscule pinhead-sized green fruit emerging from the yellow pollen centers. Barefoot, her toes squished into a full-sized tangerine rotting in the dirt.

Scrunching her face at the mushiness, she dragged her foot across the grass to clean it. Hundreds of funnel-shaped sandpit homes of the elusive doodlebug surrounded the tree's trunk. Heather poked her finger and dug into one depression, curious to find the insect, but it dug deeper, faster than her. She plucked a fluffy dandelion and held it up to big sister. Jamie puffed gently so its seeds would take flight.

After showers and all dressed up, we celebrated at Jack Baker's Lobster Shanty in south Cocoa Beach. A wood-planked bridge crossed over a pond. Jamie put quarters into the fish-food machine, letting the pellets tumble into Heather's outstretched hands. She spread her fingers and dropped all in a food shower. Lengthy orange and white koi flipped their tails and dove after the sinking morsels.

The hostess led us to a table adorned with a vase of pretty daffodils. A Jimmy Buffet song played on the music system. Wide picture windows gave a panoramic view of the Banana River and the coming sunset. Our waitress set down a plate of sugar-dusted corn fritters ladled fresh from the deep fryer. Delicious!

Though unusual for us to pray in public, but out of our immense gratitude, we joined hands as a family and gave thanks for Heather. We splurged and ordered conch fritters and rock shrimp. Shared slices of Key lime pie, chocolate cake, and scoops of coconut ice cream filled us to the brim. A few after-dinner mints, and we headed back home under a moonlit sky.

On a crisp mid-March morning, I put on my sunglasses and buckled Tony and Heather into the back seat for the four-hour drive north to Nemours for a preoperative planning appointment. They each sat by a window, a basket of toys and books stashed between. Watching the road, I couldn't see Heather's fingers "talking," so Tony spoke her signed words.

Vision wasn't needed to understand her airway. I could hear dry mucous whistles or wet gurgles. Heather would cough if prompted. Otherwise she didn't seem to feel the sensations that warned of the necessity. Dry whistle breathing was remedied by three cc plastic "fishes" about the size of a lipstick. Each contained sterile saline solution. I'd snap the cap off one and toss it to Heather.

Heather had the dexterity to squirt the saline fluid into her trach all by herself. Physiologically the liquid stream stimulated a strong cough, the forcefulness ridded her of the obstruction. Out of pure mischief, sometimes instead of tossing, I'd pop open a fish and give a fast squeeze to shoot a stream at my unsuspecting youngsters. They laughed at the antic every time.

Arriving safely in Jacksonville and onto the office, Dr. Maddern greeted us with a warm smile. "Heather looks good. She gained weight," he said. Weight gain was a gauge to judge the health of the lungs. Too unhealthy, and a child is unlikely to grow. He proceeded with his medical examination, more questions, more explanations.

He said to plan on staying a week or two. Until he incised the scarring, he wouldn't know whether her trachea would need an anterior or posterior graft or both. Keeping her asleep under heavy sedation on the ventilator for several days was a possibility. "There is an opening on the surgical schedule for Monday, April 23. If you haven't any conflicts, we'll do the airway reconstructive LTP (laryngotracheoplasty) then." He expressed his well-wishes.

Tony scrambled down the hall and raced Heather to the elevator. Once inside, he pushed the door-close button. Getting off on the first floor, Heather grabbed my hand and pulled me toward the gift shop. "Candy?" Heather signed, touching her extended index finger to her cheek.

"How about fruit?" I asked.

"Please, Mom, for the car ride," Tony begged. They each picked out three treats. I chose bubble gum and iced tea for the long drive. Holding their own packages, my two youngest dawdled, distracted by something every minute or so as we walked across the lobby to make a reservation at the Pavilion Inn. The hotel clerk printed out the confirmation. He recommended bringing along a microwave as there wasn't one in the room.

"Thanks for the suggestion," I replied. Eating something warm, other than cold cuts out of a cooler for days on end would be nice. We'd prepare for a two-week watchful vigil. There was a possibility of keeping Heather sedated and on a ventilator with a drug-induced paralysis to keep her still while the graft rooted in. A longer stay was possible if something went wrong.

Risk goes along with any surgery. Death is always a possibility. In case that disaster happened, Jim and I wanted Heather baptized. We couldn't proceed when she was a foster child, not yet adopted. Maria and Jessica drove down for the ceremony. Soon after their arrival, we took a jaunt to the beach. From my tote bag, I pulled out sunscreen. Tony whined in protest. Jamie and Jessica's friendship flourished as though they'd never been apart.

We strolled along the damp sand where the remnants of the incoming waves roll in. An eddy eroded a foot-high ledge. Thumb-size juvenile pompanos raced along its border and escaped in the retreating waters. Heather poked at some periwinkle shells. Her eyeglasses slid off and disappeared with the pompano. Nothing to rectify it; they were gone.

A great blue heron strutted, poised to steal bait from a fisherman's bucket. Jamie stepped into its sand print. The bird's foot was longer than hers. All three girls played hopscotch over clear chubby jellyfish, stayed clear of any vibrant blue Portuguese man-of-war and its long stinging tentacles.

An approaching policeman startled us. I'd never seen one on the beach before. "Excuse me, ma'am. No swimming; big fish are near the shore," he said.

"What kind of fish?" asked Jessica.

"Shhh, sharks; don't tell anybody," he answered and continued on.

At church the next day, we snapped photos of Maria and her special godchild. Too big for the family baptismal gown, Heather wore my mother's hand-stitched first communion dress. Antique ivory lace hung mid-calf, with matching veil covering most of Heather's pretty brown hair, cut pixie-style, a little girl, no longer a baby.

Unsure about the unfamiliar formalities, Heather hooked her arm around Maria's. At the sound of the priest's voice, Heather shifted her attention to him. I stood and rested my hand atop Tony's head to keep him quiet. Jim read a passage from the Bible. The priest recited more prayers before anointing Heather with the sign of the cross. Maria lit the baptismal candle. Calm contemplation settled among us as the ceremony ended.

"Maybe next time, Heather will be talking with spoken words," Jim said in hopeful expectation when it came to exchanging good-byes.

Later that afternoon we took our children on a boat ride. Crab buoys floated on the river and were tethered by a rope to a wire trap resting on the bottom. Jim steered his way through, carefully avoiding the Styrofoam balls that sometimes faded into the river. If the motor's spinning prop snagged a rope, it would entwine the blades, jerking the motor's propeller to a stop.

We were motoring up to the southern tip of Merritt Island to a famed dragon sculpture and its hatchlings guarding the waters. The Indian River is salty from ocean water ingressing through the inlets. Heather sat on the bow seat next to me. She wore a life jacket—not likely to protect her if she fell overboard—floating chest up, head tilted back, her trach would still probably take water into her lungs.

The river's surface shone glassy and smooth with gentle ripples. Ten feet in front of us, launching like a rocket from a submarine, an immense and powerful slate-colored bottle-nose dolphin shot vertically into the sky. Its body glistened in the sunlight. Drops of water showered behind like spent propellant fuel.

"What was that?" Jim exclaimed, in awe of the creature's majesty. "Guess he thought straight up was best to avoid us."

"Or he wanted to launch out of the water to get a look at Heather! Maybe her trach breathing sounds like a dolphin's blowhole."

St. Patrick's Day ushered in the final stretch of our journey to the end of the rainbow. In thirty-seven days Heather would have the laryngotracheoplasty, and we'd discover what the leprechauns had tucked into their treasure pot. Would there be audible words, giggles, and sobs? Cannonballing off a rope into an icy spring? Snorkeling amidst the splendor of Molasses Reef to watch its graceful, spotted eagle rays? Or would Heather be forever confined to the water's opaque surface and the sight of an occasional flying fish? Would sudden death always haunt us?

The pot might yield a different sort of wealth—a future molded by muteness and trach- dependence, yet full of promise. If some doors slammed shut, others would surely remain wide open. But how grand if Heather were to have a voice!

No matter what, she would have language. She was quickly mastering signing while we struggled to keep up. Sign language had disadvantages. Small moving fingers are impossible to see when darkness falls, or from another room, or if she is standing behind you.

Heather let nothing hinder her. One of her favorite adept ways of getting our attention or expressing appreciation or emotion in combination with other gestures was not appropriate in the hushed environment of a school spelling bee.

Jamie continued to spell each word correctly, as erring students were dismissed by the judge one at a time. Only two other competitors remained on stage with Jamie. To acknowledge her sister, Heather lowered her chin and sounded her loud blasts and following sputters. Every head turned to see the trumpeting elephant. Feeling a little embarrassed and in case more was to follow, I took Heather by the hand and exited quickly, missing the finale. Jamie finished as second best.

Early afternoon, Sunday, April 22, we departed for Jacksonville. The pivotal and potentially life-changing operation would soon happen. Our local pediatrician had already cleared her for surgery. The kids stood at the hospital hotel room window mesmerized by the bustling river traffic churning the water. "But I wanted to see the trains," Tony remarked.

"Oops, sorry, I forgot to request a room with a view of the trains. Maybe tomorrow the desk clerk will let us switch."

Jim had already hauled in the luggage and three cartloads that included a microwave, an eighty-gallon cooler, and non-refrigerated groceries that we stacked along a wall. He left to buy fresh milk and ice at a nearby market.

"Storm's coming. I hope Dad returns soon," Jamie said, observing a quick change in weather. Threatening black clouds blanketed the horizon. Winds picked up. Howling gusts made the whitecaps spill their froth. Hours seemed to pass.

"Rain fell in sheets, blinding at times," Jim said. His clothes were drenched. "Traffic ceased moving as soon as I drove onto the bridge. No forward motion, not an inch. Big chunks of hail pummeled the van. Stuck on the midpoint of the bridge in all the mess for over twenty minutes.

"I'm glad Dad didn't get blown off into the river," Tony said, his voice quivering at the possibility.

The next morning began the ushering in of changing possibilities. Entering the main lobby of Wolfson Children's Hospital, there was a bronzed rendering of the letter Morris David Wolfson wrote to his family of three daughters and five sons: "I hope that you boys who live after me will make sure that all persons affiliated with this clinic…have no prejudices as to race, creed, or color, and will consecrate themselves to the task of giving relief to the young that may pass through these portals. . . ."

An aide showed us to the playroom dedicated to children awaiting surgery. The colorful retreat was an arcade fantasy come true. Jamie and Tony flipped the paddles on pinball games that they could play endlessly without ever inserting a quarter. Heather wiggled into an oversized bean-bag chair before sidling over to a friendly art teacher and her table of paints. Jim and I kept watch and didn't talk about anything; too many fears might start tumbling out.

Thirty minutes before surgery, a nurse showed us to a smaller more private area, where a Peter Pan movie showed on the TV. Minutes crawled by. When I heard my mother's voice, I relaxed a smidgen. Heather's nose crinkled, and the corners of her mouth turned up into a straight-line smile. She ran to greet her Grandy and got busy sifting through her purse until she found a lipstick and powder.

The door opened again, and in walked Dr. Maddern, exuding poise and jovial confidence, diligently earned through many years of dedicated study and experience. An amused Dr. Maddern looked on as my mom applied make-up to her special granddaughter. "Heather looks as if she's enjoying herself," he said, grinning.

"She likes her Grandy," I said.

"When did you get into town?" he asked my mom.

"A few minutes ago," Mom answered. "The others arrived yesterday."

After Jim recounted his story of being caught in the storm, the doctor told one of his own, adding gestures and expressions specifically to entertain Heather. "A tree fell on our house," he said, "but there wasn't much damage."

"What happens now?" Jim asked.

"A nurse will give her a sedative to make her sleepy. Depending on how complicated the airway repair procedure is, the operation should take about three hours. Halfway through, someone will apprise you on how we are proceeding."

Heather looked up at him, touching her fingertips to her chin, letting her hand drop forward until it was parallel to the floor, palm up. "That's the sign for *thanks*," I said.

"I know," he replied.

Jim gave him a hearty handshake, and so did I. The gestures seemed an understated expression of our gratefulness. Airway surgery is tricky business, especially for a child with Heather's history. We prayed all would be well.

"He's a nice man," I said to Mom.

"And he looked rested," she commented. "I'm glad I arrived in time to meet him."

A nurse pointed to a stack of child-sized hospital gowns. Jim changed Heather into a soft flannel one printed with bright cartoon characters. Heather tapped her fingers on a tawny lion, her expression inquiring how to form the sign for the word. Jim swept his open right hand back from his forehead creating a visual image of a mane.

Looking at Jim, my mom, Jamie, and Tony, and the love that poured out to Heather, and the love she shone back to us, I thought of the wooden plaque that hung in our living room. It was a gift from Mark and Celeste. The plaque displayed a crucifix with a little girl kneeling in prayer before it. Inscribed beneath were the words, "God's Gift to the Gigantis: Heather."

CHAPTER 19]
SURGERY

Gloved and gowned figures moved about, preparing the operating room. An assistant, a scrub tech, and two circulating nurses opened surgical packs, maintaining sterile technique while arranging dozens of instruments. The anesthesiologist checked his life-sustaining machines and supplies. He and Dr. Maddern would work in close partnership for Heather's safety.

"It's time," a nurse murmured, interrupting our children's play. She read aloud Heather's identification bracelet and verified that it matched pre-surgery paperwork and that all of the checklist had been completed. Mom voiced warm encouragement and hugged each of us. She took hold of Jamie's and Tony's hands, and the three of them left for a day of exploring the Museum of Science and History and the local zoo.

"Thanks Mom," I said.

"Excuse me," I said to the nurse. "Please post this on the front of her chart." On cardstock paper I'd written in bright marker this information: "Heather is mute. She is physically unable to talk and uses sign language to communicate. Her hearing is good."

"No problem. I'll tell everybody in the surgical suite and in the recovery room too," she assured me.

"Are you taking her back now?" Jim asked.

"Yes, but both of you are coming along," she said. "Children remain calm and happy if parents tend to them until the anesthesia casts its spell."

The kind nurse escorted us to the induction room. She instructed me to sit in a special chair with Heather on my lap. Alongside me, she pulled a seat for Jim. Dr. Davis, the anesthesiologist, introduced himself and gave Heather a small toy— a blue plastic moose no bigger than a thumb, a gesture that captured her imagination.

"Jim, would you assist me?" the doctor asked, handing over the anesthetic line and guiding Jim how to direct the sleeping gas so Heather would breathe it. Lighthearted banter about the moose distracted our brave little girl. After a few moments, she went limp in my arms. Her lungs moved air easily without extra muscling or congestion. Dr. Davis and the nurse took over.

Their procedural wisdom thwarted any crying—and for Heather, its sequel of emotionally triggered labored breathing, gurgles and plugs. It avoided fear induced by a stranger escorting a child away from the parents, and prevented fright triggered by the unusual happenings as Jim and I were involved.

A volunteer showed us to the waiting area. I felt like a pot boiled dry, yet bubbling over with joyful anticipation, all at the same time. Perhaps, maybe, just maybe, Dr. Maddern would surgically gift Heather with a patent healthy airway, and she would talk. Lacking access to a pool to ease my nerves, a brisk walk would suffice. Jim and I traversed the corridor that led past the medical offices to the hotel.

"Would you reassign us a room with a view of the passing cargo trains? My son loves watching them." Jim inquired. The desk clerk obliged. Busying ourselves with relocating the luggage and personal deli to the new room, we gained the illusion of time passing more quickly. Jim and I stumbled upon a small chapel and knelt in prayer.

The operating room's white walls and gray floors sparkled with cleanliness. Large rectangular lights filled the ceiling. Two adjustable round ones hung suspended directly over the operating table. A scrub tech slipped sterile covers over the handles so the beams could be readjusted without breaking the sterility of the surgical field. An assistant chose a compact disc to play muted rock-and-roll as they worked.

9:30 a.m. Surgery, examining the airways

A light sedative dripped through an IV into a vein in Heather's left hand. Light anesthesia, so she could continue to breathe naturally through the trach. Maddern inserted the smooth metal examining blade of a laryngoscope into her mouth. He peered down at her vocal cords, which look like taut but flexible bands of polished pearl. Light anesthesia let there be a possibility of their moving and a better understanding of their structure, before deeper anesthesia vanquished them to immobility. Heather's vocal cords were scarred, victims of trauma from ventilators and endotracheal tubes. Maddern could not ascertain whether their lack of movement was from never being used or that they were paralyzed.

He withdrew the laryngoscope and passed a bronchoscope that expanded his view to include the lower airways. The examining device displayed a simultaneous image on a television screen. Still pictures and video film recorded the findings. The team's mood was subdued and serious but joyous. The superstars played with a private confidence in their ability to brighten a child's future.

9:50 a.m. Surgery, draping and surgical airway

Dr. Davis positioned an egg-crate shaped foam pad under Heather's upper torso. He ran a strip of tape across her closed eyes to keep them shut and prevent injury. The circulating nurse removed Heather's gown. Monitors were placed. A screen displayed continuously her EKG, oxygen and carbon-dioxide levels, heart and respiratory rates, for all to observe. The nurse painted Heather's chest with an antiseptic iodine solution from chin to navel.

Maddern pulled the trach out of the breathing hole in her neck and replaced it with a flexible wire-reinforced surgical airway that he sutured in place. The room was too warm for the heavily attired team but just right for Heather's bare skin. A stack of blue sterile towels disappeared one by one as Maddern draped them over her body until only a narrow section of chest was exposed.

Dr. Davis turned on the Bair Hugger, a machine that circulates warm air beneath a patient. Along with all her vital functions, he'd monitor her temperature readings. He deepened the anesthesia.

Now that Heather was covered and warmed, an assistant turned down the air conditioner's thermostat for the comfort of the surgical team.

10:05 a.m. Surgery, incising the right chest.

Dr. Maddern delicately incised skin layers and deeper into her right chest. After a few minutes her sixth and seventh ribs glistened under the bright lights. He harvested a two-by-four centimeter cartilagine rib segment and wrapped it in saline-soaked gauze. To test for an inadvertent lung puncture, Dr. Davis gently increased the inflation of Heather's lungs. The greater pressure would cause any leakage of air to visibly bubble up through the fluids pooling in the gaping wound. There were none, and the site was closed.

A scrub nurse stripped off the soiled surgical drapes and towels. She replaced them with fresh ones arranging them strategically for the next stage, stapling them into position. A small square of Heather's neck skin remained visible.

10:25 a.m. Surgery, incising the neck.

Beneath the team's surgical masks that covered the nose and mouth, exhaled breath condensed into a fine mist and drifted upward through the gap, leaving behind tiny beads of moisture clinging to everyone's eyelashes and brows.

Dr. Maddern cut a horizontal incision through the skin of her neck. He spread the edges with a retractor. He then began cutting in the opposite direction—a delicate vertical incising of tissues, avoiding arteries and nerves, until he reached the damaged larynx (voice box). As he progressed, he gently touched an electrically heated Bovie tip to bleeding vessels to cauterize them, staunching the flow. Each touch sent out a whiff of burnt flesh. An assistant dabbed away any remnant trickling blood lest it drip down her windpipe and into the lungs and cause pneumonia.

Maddern cut into the troublesome scarring with a pair of Metzenbaum scissors and continued with a razor-sharp number 15 scalpel. He split the larynx and upper trachea vertically, exposing the scarred structures. Studying all he saw, he determined that Heather would need an eight-by-twenty millimeter anterior graft but nothing posteriorly.

At this point, a circulating nurse phoned the waiting room and informed us of the plan. She said all was well, and we felt grateful.

Readying the trachea to receive the enlarging graft, Dr. Maddern used a cutting needle threaded with a dissolvable suture and pierced the right tracheal edge. He pulled the needle through and released it, still gripped by a needle holder, letting it dangle down Heather's draped neck. Soon he'd attached a total of twelve weighted sutures: six hung from the right side, and six from the left. An assistant suctioned the operative site of secretions to keep all visible. Several ccs of blood-tinged fluid flowed through clear tubing into a collection canister.

11:00 a.m. Surgery, Shaping the graft.

Dr. Maddern used a scalpel to sculpt the harvested rib graft into a flattened ellipse. He beveled the edges so that when it was attached, it wouldn't collapse into the tracheal lumen.

Maddern's deft hands whittled away a portion of a plastic T-tube, modifying the bottom of the device to support the grafted airway during healing. Satisfied, he positioned the long part of the T-tube like a vertical straw inside the trachea.

Just above, forceps suspended the anterior cartilagine graft like a motionless kite. One by one Maddern pierced the graft with each of the waiting dangling needles, setting them at calculated dangles. Meticulously, he pulled each fragment tighter, lowering the graft painstakingly slowly until it was snug in its place. The graft opened up her scarred airway.

After tightening the last of the stiches, he flexed Heather's neck to check for buckling or separation of the graft. He positioned a short drainage tube into the wound to keep a small tract open when he stitched it closed. Otherwise, unable to escape, air and blood gets trapped within the tissues and pressure the airway, narrowing its diameter and hindering breathing.

12:25 p.m. Surgery, ending anesthesia and waking up Heather

Dr. Davis removed the flexible airway from the tracheotomy hole and reinserted a Shiley trach. Maddern used the laryngoscope to take a last look through Heather's mouth to make sure all was as it should be with the T-tube stent in place.

After two hours and fifty-five minutes, thirty-nine needles, and dozens of sponges, the operation was finished. Davis reversed the anesthesia, and Heather woke up. They moved her to the recovery area to be monitored by nurses adept at immediate postoperative care.

I looked up from page eight of my book to see Dr. Maddern smiling at us. "It went fine," he said, going on to describe everything he'd done. "She can't talk yet, with the T-tube stent in place. There's not enough room for air to go around it." He drew a diagram so we'd understand. "She could go home as early as Friday."

Jim and I tried to convey the depths of our gratitude. Our expression of thanks seemed woefully inadequate. "How long until she will be in recovery?" Jim asked.

"Maybe an hour more."

"That'll run close to the shift change. They'll stall on moving her to PICU, push it off onto the arriving evening nurses," I said.

"You know the drill," he replied.

"I guess we'll go get a sandwich."

Neither Jim or I had eaten all day. Maybe a meal would boost our energy. We wandered over to the coffee shop and ordered a couple of hoagies. Fearing that maybe they would transfer her sooner than anticipated; we finished quickly and walked to PICU to wait for Heather's arrival.

Each intensive-care patient had a private room. The inner wall was constructed of glass and was rotated toward the nurses' work area, so they could observe. A curtain could be pulled for privacy. Out of long established habit, I located the oxygen, suction, and resuscitative supplies and confirmed that they worked. Jim placed the emergency bag in close reach.

Elevator doors clanked open, and a rolling crib rattled down the hall. We scrambled to meet it. In her right hand, Heather clutched the little moose. Dr. Davis must have placed it in her hand at the conclusion of his after-surgery monitoring. Heather's eyes opened, and some silent crying began.

"Remember about the *owies*. How at first it would hurt when Dr. Maddern fixed your airway. It will get all better," I promised. "Then we'll throw away your trach. You'll breathe through your nose, and get to talk, and go swimming!"

The nurse disconnected Heather from the rolling oxygen tank and portable monitors, reconnecting her to the ones in the room. Painkillers made Heather dopey, so she dozed off.

At dusk Mom arrived with Jamie and Tony. Heather perked up at the sound of her sister and brother and Grandy talking. Jamie flipped channels with the TV's remote control. Tony climbed right into the crib to comfort and amuse his little sister with his comic ways. Their presence seemed as important as the narcotic dripping into her vein. Heather tendered a feeble smile and eased herself up into a sitting position.

"Drink please," she signed with her fingers. A nurse brought some orange Gatorade. Heather grasped the cup, but pushed it toward my mom.

"No thanks, it's for you honey," my mom said. Heather insisted and tremulously lifted the cup to her grandmother's lips before drinking some herself. She snuggled up with her favorite stuffed animal, Lamby. Everyone except me headed off to the hotel. The kids blew kisses.

I tipped back the sleeper chair and settled in. I shut my eyes, though my ears stayed tuned to the sound of Heather's breathing. I suctioned her when needed, never inserting the catheter past the near end of the trach tube.

The long night seemed a time warp, a twilight zone where alarms and the sound of moving, living air were all that mattered. At last the sun glinted through the curtains. Dr. Maddern stopped in and examined Heather on his morning rounds. Jim relieved me. One of us tended to Heather at all times. We had more at stake than the nurses on duty and were more alert to the potential for dire complications.

Mom departed with Jamie and Tony to visit the Cummer Museum of Art and its gardens. I slipped into the hotel bed and slept deeply. Mid-afternoon, after a refreshing shower and eating a bowl of warmed-up Brunswick stew, I joined Jim at Heather's cribside.

"She's really agitated and refuses to eat or drink," he said. "The nurse injected an extra dose of morphine into the IV." Jim suggested that I stretch out in the reclining chair. He gathered Heather up and placed her on my chest. I enfolded her into my arms. Her poor belly was taut from accumulated gas. Sleepy intestines not moving flatus along were a side-effect of the general anesthesia.

"She feels warm," I remarked.

"She's running a mild fever. Antibiotics have already been started," Jim said.

As I comforted my little girl, an unnamed energy seemed to flow from my being to hers—restoring her and tiring me. We both fell asleep. Jim remained awake, seated, quietly watching over us, no television. Praying.

Later that evening, Dr. Maddern pulled the seepage drains out of Heather's neck and chest, and bandaged the wounds. "Get her walking in the hallway. Moving around will help her pass the gas and encourages greater lung expansion. Both aid in reducing fever and help to prevent pneumonia."

Jim coaxed Heather to ease up to a stand. Slowly she proceeded down the corridor, stopping at doorways to peek in on other children. Near the turnaround, beloved Betsey breezed in toting a bouquet of floating balloons and two giant bags stuffed with toys. She plopped down on the floor next to Heather. The nurse's dark hair bounced with her animated talk. Heather lifted her hand and rested it on the young woman's shoulder. Toys came tumbling out. Jim tied the balloons to the rolling IV pole. For over an hour we played right there. No one was in a hurry to return to the room.

Wednesday morning the dressings came off, leaving her neck and chest incisions open to air. Heather no longer needed morphine. Tylenol with codeine administered by a spoon eased her pain. Her belly softened. Feeling better, boredom ensued. Approved for a trip to the playroom, plentiful activities entertained us until it closed. Afterward, Heather roamed up and down the hallway. The emergency bag followed behind.

Day four, Heather still refused to eat. Dr. Maddern's frustration peaked. "Get any of her favorites. I don't care what: junk food, McDonald's," he suggested. The Golden Arches and its french fries did the trick. She ate all of a small order.

Dr. Maddern explained the changing nuances to her care. Looking like a tacky bow tie, layers of gauze were folded under and over the side flanges of her trach to cushion the healing incision in her neck. "The T-tube stent crowds her airway. It increases the resistance felt during a trach change. Hold on to the T-protrusion so that the stent is not pulled out when removing the old trach, or pushed in when inserting a new one," he warned. "Don't use the Passy-Muir® speaking valve. It won't work. It's too crowded for air to pass through her vocal cords. Not until after she comes back and has the stent removed."

The next morning, Dr. Maddern gave the okay for Heather to go home. Amazing, the dream of Heather having a voice had moved from a whimsical thought to an actual possibility. Jim and I hoped that she would not develop any wound infections, which could attack the rooting in of the graft, or impact the healing of the incisions in her chest and neck.

Before we left for home, we stopped by his clinic. A mother of a child with a tracheotomy had some fears and wished to ask us a few questions.

Ann Widick Giganti

Laryngotracheoplasty, LTP graphics courtesy of Nemours
Airway reconstruction with a rib cartilage graft

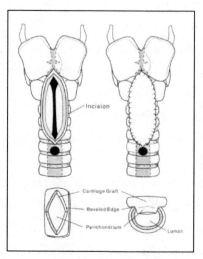

Relationship of incised trachea and
harvested rib cartilage graft

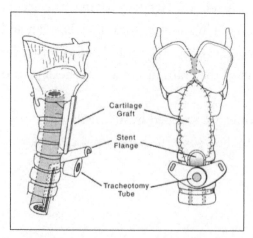

Side view showing relationship of supporting
stent and tracheotomy tube

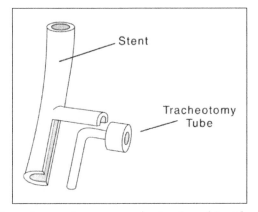

How the tracheotomy tube is placed inside the
modified T-tube stent

CHAPTER 20] SWEET SUCCESS

Two weeks later, it was a school holiday. My sister's two sons were spending the day with us. They both found Heather's muteness confusing. Tony thought it everyday normal. So normal that he'd concluded that all babies are born into this world with a trach in the neck.

Because of her recent surgery, Heather kept to the confines of the house and back porch. She felt only brief twinges of pain unless she bumped into something. She'd dressed herself in rose sweatpants and a pink cotton shirt. On her head, the happy child wore her favorite yellow knitted cap, even on the warm day. Her chestnut-colored hair bounced a trifle and hung to just below her shoulders. Bopping about, her pink-rimmed glasses slid down her nose. Her face broadcast large smiles and impish dimples.

Cousin Daniel, who was about Heather's same age, suddenly grabbed hold of Heather around her chest and wouldn't let go.

"Don't hug her so tight. Her ribs have an *owie*." I scolded him.

"She never talks. I did it on purpose so maybe she'd holler and make some noise," Daniel replied.

I tried explaining about her muteness and how after one more quick surgery, she might have a voice. "Maybe she'll babble like a baby, and the cousins can help teach her to talk. Or maybe, her first spoken words will be 'Let's go out to Pizza Hut.'" An acquaintance I'd made, her son's first spoken words after trach removal happened to be the pizza for dinner request.

"Aunt Ann, I used sign language when I was small. One day I woke up talking. Heather will too." Six-year-old Bryan concocted a fiction.

Our hang-out-together days always began with a basket of art supplies and booklets on how to draw sea creatures or cartoon characters. The cousins scavenged through and retrieved their own sketch books.

"Bumblebee, the tuna. I'll draw him," Tony said.

"Raisin," Daniel said.

"Huh?" Bryan asked, glancing at his brother with a puzzled expression.

"There's a raisin squished in my booklet," Daniel announced. "Looks like a dried bug."

Jamie chose to draw Scooby. Heather selected fat crayons and a mermaid coloring book. Bryan penciled an intricate octopus by drawing a light-bulb shape to fashion its head and vague pipe-cleaner legs that he strengthened and shaded.

With an eraser Daniel sharpened the square corners of the menacing teeth of his killer whale. When satisfied, they signed and dated their drawings before wandering out to the backyard for imaginative play.

Along came the month of June. We trekked back to the hospital for Dr. Maddern to attempt the removal of the T-tube stent. If the cartilagine graft had successfully healed and attached itself to her trachea, she'd have an open, patent airway. Before her surgery, we played arcade games in the waiting area until a nurse escorted us back to the holding room. I again held Heather until she drifted into anesthesia-induced sleep. Jim did his part, holding the line of flowing anesthetic gas.

In the operating room, Maddern inserted the fiberoptic scope to examine the full length of her trachea. One soft fleshy mound of scar tissue reared its head near the trach opening. Utilizing the aiming beam of the laser, with a punch of his finger, a concentrated ray of light fired, vaporizing the pesky granuloma.

Dr. Maddern ambled into the waiting area still wearing his surgical scrubs. "The T-tube stent is out. I am very pleased with how well the graft has healed. Her airway is free of scarring and wide open. Breath flowing through her unused vocal cords will wake them up and get them moving and minimize any new formation of granulomas." The more he talked, the more he boosted our hope for an improvement in Heather's present health and future possibilities.

Once the transport nurse moved Heather and settled her into a private room on the pediatric floor, Maddern came back around. He handed me a speaking valve, and reviewed the risks associated with using it, the biggest being suffocation. A reconstructed airway could narrow for many reasons and obstruct breathing, or the device might malfunction. Poor coordination would preclude Heather's little fingers from plucking it off. It has that built-in pop-off safety feature, but Heather's muscles were still too weak to cough and eject it.

"Go ahead," Dr. Maddern urged.

"Cross our fingers," I said, afraid that the long anticipated stupendous moment was me dreaming or maybe a mirage.

Maddern watched as I gingerly positioned the device onto the trach. Heather inhaled a breath through its one-way flap. On exhalation the valve closed, not bulging. It easily redirected exhaling breath outward around the trach tube resting inside her trachea and onward through her vocal cords, flowing out her mouth and nose. "Maaaa," slipped out without any conscious effort on her part.

"Did you hear that?" Maddern exclaimed. Unrestrained enthusiasm leapt his voice ten notches, full of life.

I smiled, relieved it hadn't been my imagination.

Rapidly as a chameleon changes colors, Heather's happy countenance switched to fright. She pursed her lips tight and kept them that way, willing them to stitch together. The sensation of creating sound scared her, so it seemed.

"Keep the valve on. Have her breathe through the Passy-Muir® whenever she's awake. Take it off for sleeping." Dr. Maddern insisted on meticulous and continuous observation of her breathing while using the device.

Inhaling through the valve and exhaling out her nose proved easy for her. As instructed, after a couple of weeks, we replaced her tracheotomy tube with one of a smaller diameter. Greater volumes of air could exit around a narrower tube.

Boy oh boy, did we long to hear her voice! But no matter how much we coaxed, adorable Heather would let no sound slip out her lips: not a single vowel, nor even giggles or sobs. She kept her mouth resolutely zipped closed with psychologically manufactured gorilla-strength impenetrable stitches.

Fear loomed. Perhaps she wasn't afraid? Maybe her vocal cords didn't move, rendering her unable to form sounds. Maybe for Heather the mechanics of making speech seemed unfathomable.

Patience, remember patience, but we didn't want to be patient. Perhaps concentrating on a new way to breathe occupied all of her energies, and spoken language would follow. There was another big milestone to reach: inhaling through her nose instead of the neck. Was she strong enough?

Due to the increase in the length of the airway, breathing in from the nose to the lungs increases the work of breathing three-fold compared to breathing in through the neck. To build up her muscle strength and let her sneak a little air in through her nose, we placed tape over one-fourth of the speaking-valve opening.

Jim or I kept our eyes on her, every second, always observing for signs of respiratory distress or insufficient oxygenation. We kept increasing the amount of taping until we covered over the entire speaking valve, causing her to inhale and exhale each breath solely through her nose or mouth.

No verbal sounds had slipped out of Heather since that first chance utterance in the hospital. Three weeks passed. Four weeks passed. The month of July rolled in, hot and muggy. Even all of the day of her third birthday, she kept her lips pressed together.

We celebrated her birthday with a cook-out. Jamie and Heather both wore pretty flowered dresses. Guests were arriving, and we stood in the shade of an oak tree in the front yard. We saw my father cruising down our avenue in his newest automobile, tailed by a police car. The driveway was full so Dad veered his vehicle onto the grass lawn and parked. He opened his door, stood up, and began walking our way, seemingly oblivious to the slowing patrol vehicle.

"Fritz, were you driving too fast?" Jim asked.

"Not me," Dad protested. "Why?"

Jim gestured toward the officer parking his vehicle.

The officer got out and strode purposefully toward us. "Ma'am, what's going on here?" he questioned sternly, his face gruff.

"A party for my daughter's third birthday."

"Someone dialed the 911 emergency number. The dispatcher only heard rough breathing," he said.

"My youngest daughter is mute. She has a trach. She can't make verbal sounds. Her breathing makes a lot of turbulent noise. Maybe she was playing with the phone," I said and called her over.

Heather formed the signs for *me* (a flat hand pat on the chest) and *phone* (partially closed fist with thumb and pinky extended, held to the ear like a phone) and the finger movements for the word *play*.

"Just the same, I must look through your house," he replied.

Jim accompanied the officer as he performed a cursory search of each room. I stayed outside with Dad and Heather. Mr. Officer said little, bid us good day, and departed.

The festivities resumed.

Out back at the picnic table, Jim layered salt and ice in the ice-cream churn. People took turns with the hand-cranking. Stylishly attired as usual, my mom set down a fancy package. Heather fumbled with its wrapping paper. Jamie assisted by enclosing Heather's fingers in hers and ripping a corner. Inside were some children's books. More gift opening. Hamburgers. Corn on the cob. Delicious.

Mom brought out her home-baked lemon-frosted cake dotted with maraschino cherries. Granddaddy Fritz struck a match and lit three candles. Heather clapped with delight. All sang "Happy Birthday" and hoped that Heather's voice would join the chorus at its next rendition. Dad spooned on scoops of rich hand-cranked vanilla ice cream onto the cake slices. As the evening slowed, many of us strolled the short walk to Riverside Park and watched the sunset.

Stoic anticipation. Luckily the next ten days flew by until the epitome of the voice search saga loomed less than twenty hours into the future. We travelled to Jacksonville and checked into the Pavilion Inn.

Two things could happen. The outcome would be either stupendous or really bad. After freeing Heather's trachea of its lifelong tracheotomy tube companion, we'd throw away the trach tube. Or the graft would fail, and Heather's airway would collapse into itself.

Optimism woke us before the alarm sounded. There was no surgery, so Heather had stayed with us in the hotel room. We dressed and hurried to the PICU. In case something went wrong, the removal would transpire there. Adrenalin surged awaiting Maddern's arrival. To busy ourselves, Jim folded paper into airplanes for the kids to toss around the room. I prayed to God and the Holy Spirit and hoped that any guardian angels hovering in the upper corners of the room would increase their watchfulness.

At 9:06 a.m. on July 31, 1990, Dr. Maddern stepped into the room, exuding confidence. "I see everyone is having fun here," he said, surveying the fleet of aircraft. Acting as master of ceremonies, he spoke slowly, drawing out his words for dramatic effect. "At last the moment we have all been waiting for." He snipped the cloth ties that secured Heather's trach. With a gentle tug, he pulled the tube out.

We listened, keen on hearing the high-pitched whistles of airway collapse or the deafening silence of complete obstruction. We stared, mesmerized, searching for telltale signs of respiratory distress and its incipient dusky pallor.

Success! Sweet, blessed air flowed through Heather's nose and mouth without aid for the first time in her three years of life. Her face glowed with a happy radiance and a nonstop smile.

Dr. Bruce Robert Maddern stood tall, grinning, hazel eyes sparkling. Giddy with joy, we shared the indescribable euphoria of living a miracle.

Heather patted her chest with the palm of her hand for "me" and moved both arms in breaststroke motions, laughing with her whole body.

"Yes, you can swim! And snorkel, and even sail across the ocean to the Bahamas," Jim said, equally ecstatic.

Exuberant Heather grabbed our hands and marched us on a parade through the hallways, showering all with her happy spirit, proudly pointing to her trachless neck. A colorful bandage covered the remnant hole. Staff cheered and offered a confetti of well-wishes.

She stayed in PICU for several days. Cardiorespiratory and oxygen saturation machines stuck to her, ceaselessly monitoring for a failing airway. Dulled from years of housing a tube, nerve endings in Heather's airway lacked a normal sensitivity to irritants, so there was no reflex coughing. Whenever necessary, we'd have to remind her to cough until the critical sense redeveloped.

While still in the hospital and its ready assistance, Jim wanted to challenge Heather with anything that might precipitate trouble. He walked her up and down stairwells. He put her through her usual daily activities. We brainstormed and came up with some challenging exercise routines. Heather's reconstructed anatomy passed all challenges.

Swimming would have to wait for the vestigial hole in her neck to heal. If her body wouldn't mend the opening, Dr. Maddern would have to surgically close it.

Our attempts at expressing our immense thankfulness to Dr. Maddern seemed woefully inadequate. Heading for home, giddiness at the miracle of trach-free Heather again consumed us. Traversing this crazy storm of meeting Heather and the clouds that followed, we'd ended up climbing over the tallest of rainbows and landed in the Leprechauns' pot of gold. Tucked in there, they'd hidden an assortment of the greatest of gifts. In there, we'd found the Voice Giver—Dr. Bruce Robert Maddern.

Heather was not utilizing his gift of voice, but she would eventually, we were quite confident. The confidence stemming from the single "maaaa" that slipped out.

In my grateful imaginings, I hoped that perhaps one day we would meet another superstar—Dr. Robin Cotton, the dedicated surgeon who'd invented the LTP airway reconstructive procedure that was changing Heather's life and ours in such wonderful ways.

FREEDOM FROM BONDAGE. Medical routines no longer gobbled up our time. Time multiplied seemingly exponentially. As instructed by Dr. Maddern, after seven days, we got rid of the portable and electrical suction machines and all other gear, including the reverberating humidifier, monitors, and alarms.

"I'm not worrying that we might need them. I've done enough worrying for several lifetimes," I said to Jim.

"I'll fret for both of us," Jim said, and made a screwy face.

Soon he fell asleep. In our double bed, the left side was Jim's, and the right was mine. He had on ragged old gym shorts and a T-shirt. Arms and legs sprawled straight out. The sharp angle of his jaw was heavily stubbled with a day's beard growth.

Quiet. Without the background noises of Heather's machinery, the night was quiet. This new quiet began to play tricks. No noise to mask anxiety, or block out fear for Heather's safety. In the middle of the night, the silence in the house seemed deafening. Still air vibrated, humming its undulating song of molecules colliding.

The ticking of the clock on my bedside table grew louder. Jim's stomach rumbled. The air-conditioning compressor cut on. Its noise was comforting. It blocked out the silent night. The AC cycled off, quiet again. The old walls of the house creaked. Outside the wind bustled a palm frond and scratched it against the window.

Maybe running the AC fan continually until daybreak would assist with this transition from a backdrop cacophony of medical equipment to silence. Get up and flip on the thermostat settings, lazybones, I told myself. I stepped into the hallway and slid the switch. The constant gentle noises of the AC's central fan became my lullaby.

I suppressed any musings of her airway collapsing to the deep recesses of my mind. I yawned and stretched and rolled over onto my side. In a spell of happiness and gratitude, I fell asleep. Oblivious to the future, I thought we were done with all major surgeries, but we weren't. Heather's teenage years would again send us seeking a surgeon's cure.

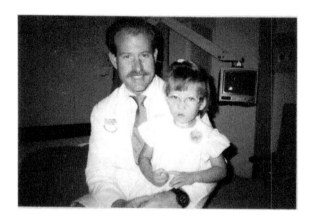

Dr. Bruce Robert Maddern, pediatric otolaryngologist.

Surgeon who performed the surgery.

Miracle day!

He just removed the tracheotomy from Heather's neck.

CHAPTER 21] EAGLE RAYS

Maybe Heather might grow up to have it all: education, self-supporting, family of her own. We'd found the Voice Giver, but she was still the voiceless child, not using the gift that she had been given. Most likely it was stubbornness. Jim and I refused to entertain the concept of any type of brain damage.

A wondrous new experience began—life with healthy Heather. Once we'd defined health for Heather as simply breathing, no expectation of purposeful movement, and most important—having us as a family. I'd come to realize that the definition of health is ambiguous and changing and is relative and unique to each personal experience. For Heather, it had progressed to include walk, run, eat, drink, be mischievous, and bestow love.

I signed her up for ballet. Readying for class, she sure looked cute, putting one leg and then the other into a pink leotard, like any other child. At the studio, Robyn, also three years old, danced next to her. They giggled and became instant friends as I did with her mom.

Open-minded Linda noticed Heather's scarred neck and the open, trach hole that sometimes bubbled mucous. She didn't ask any questions just chatted endlessly about small town stuff. The dance instructor exempted me from her no-parents present during class rule. She let me remain so I could keep a watchful eye for any breathing difficulties and to translate Heather's rudimentary sign language.

Breakthrough! The first parting of Heather's zipped lips occurred on an outing to Sebastian Inlet, a man-made cut that links the Indian River to the Atlantic Ocean. Its treacherous tides rip and curl and can ensnare and sink any boat that has an inexperienced captain.

There is a shallow cove that is protected from the inlet by a buttress of rocks. Picnic tables are scattered along its sandy shore. Jim and I relaxed in the shade of a palm tree, listening to sea-gulls squawk as they chattered in their foraging flights.

Heather couldn't swim as the vestigial hole in her neck remained. With the tide out, she chased fiddler crabs scurrying about the mud flats. Jamie and Tony skipped toward the retreating tide, minnow-dipping nets and buckets ready, scooping fingerlings trapped in the vanishing pools.

Currents washed in cool, clear, serene water, no deeper than your knees. We waded over to a line of piled-up granite boulders and climbed to a higher vantage. A drifting shadow seemed cast by a cloud darkened the waters, until its fleshy snout surfaced and blew out a fine mist. Moseying by was a manatee, as long as two bathtubs.

A half-dozen pelicans lazed on the piers. Some with their heads tucked beneath a wing. Others spread their wings to dry, end-feathers fluttering in the breeze. We strolled the concrete walkway that ran along the top of the rock jetties that jutted far into the ocean. Jim ensured Heather's steps avoided strewn, dried catfish with their venomous barbs. We peered into five-gallon buckets of salt water to see each fisherman's catch.

Heather paused on a section that had heavy grating beneath her feet instead of concrete. Mesmerized, she gazed through at the waves sloshing roughly among the rock piles. A larger

swell crashed and shot water up at Heather like a whale blowing its spout, drenching her. Laughter gushed out, even though Heather attempted to stifle its sound. Bless that wave. Bless the fun of hearing the beautiful sounds of Heather's amusement for the very first time.

Twice a week appointments with Debra, the speech therapist, began a further melting of Heather's resistance to spoken language. To reinforce learning how to manipulate the tongue to form basic sounds, Debra would dab peanut butter on Heather's upper or lower lip and have her touch it with the tip of her tongue. Another variation for learning tongue mobility to specific spots, perhaps the gum line behind her upper teeth, was to have her touch her tongue to a tuft of foam positioned there by a lollipop-like stick.

Homework involved tasks to strengthen and improve the mobility of the muscles in her tongue and cheeks. They seemed underdeveloped, a consequence of having never been used during all those months that tube feedings sustained her. Exercises included sucking thick liquids through a special straw.

Miraculous Heather forged ahead full of enthusiasm, no longer fearful of the sounds and words that she vocalized. Hearing her say "Mama" and "Dada" for the first time charmed us to the umpteenth power. Additional words followed like an avalanche. She devoted so much energy to learning spoken language that she reverted to wearing diapers for several months.

Hanging out in the waiting area at speech therapy, Heather and I befriended a woman and her foster son and daughter. She was Caucasian, and the children were black. After a session, we sometimes visited their home. I often complimented her on its spick-and-span appearance. Heather and her friend often played puzzles, though he wouldn't talk. I never asked why he could not speak.

The child missed sessions two weeks in a row. I called his foster mom to check on them. Her reply shocked me. "The caseworker removed both kids. She alleged my house was too cluttered. Nonsense. I don't think she wanted dark-skinned children living with a white mama. I'm hiring an attorney." It took about a month, but she got the children back.

November, 1990. All that was once impossible became fully achievable. Dr. Maddern brought Heather back to the operating room and surgically closed the vestigial hole in her neck. Sweet success. Uneventful healing. She could loll in a tub and submerge under bath bubbles. At my parents' pool, she'd jump into Jim's waiting arms. Swimming came to her without much effort, just frequent opportunity. At the ocean, she learned to ride waves on a boogey board.

About a year after she got her tracheotomy tube out, my dad planned an afternoon of sailing on his forty-four foot ketch, *Guffey*, named after his Aunt. He'd bought the hull for nine-hundred dollars, painted it white with a sleek blue waterline stripe. It is probably the only sailboat in the world outfitted with metal salvaged from a launch-pad demolition.

Smaller scrap metal pellets became the boat's stabilizing ballast. Long pieces of salvage pipe constructed the boom and a two-part telescopic mast, so it could pass under the bridges. Telescopic, remove a pin and the smaller diameter upper section could slide down into the lower section. With a shortened mast, he could moor the boat at home, sail along the river, or through the port to the ocean, and even cross to the Bahamas.

From my parents' dock, we all clambered on board. Heather's meandering was limited to the inside cabin or the protected seating in the cockpit. Dad motored the *Guffey* through the creeks of the Thousand Islands to reach the open river. "Grab hold of the helm," Dad told Heather. She was only a head taller than the spoked steering wheel.

"It's too big!" Heather protested. Her words emphatic, but the actual sound quiet and a little whispery.

"I'll be right beside you," Dad said. "Place your left hand at twelve o'clock, right hand at three o'clock. Hold tight; you're strong," Heather steered a straight course. Her muscular legs kept her balanced.

Winds rising, Dad took back the helm and headed into the gusts. My brothers and Jim hoisted the jib, main, and mizzen sails. Dad adjusted course until the sails stopped rippling and grew taut. Engine off. Strong winds sped us along.

The *Guffey* heeled sharply, guard rail teasing the water. Salty spray engulfed us. Each of us gripped something tightly so we didn't slide overboard. No sitting near the metal heavy boom. Shifting winds and one swing of it against your noggin would knock a person out, maybe permanently.

Nimble nephew Bryan climbed high on a rope ladder that ascended the mast and scanned the river. "Dolphins!" he shouted. The speed of the *Guffey* slicing through the river curled waves against its bow. Streamlined gray bodies streaked by us to play in the churning water. One rolled sideways to peer up at us, momentarily flashing his lighter underside. A younger one dropped off, flipped his tail, and pumped forward for a rapid return. We slapped the boat's wooden sides in appreciation, eager to prolong the mammals' frolic.

A flock of white pelicans veered toward Bird Island, a sanctuary off-limits to people. Through binoculars Mom spotted ibises, herons, and a few roseate spoonbills. At dusk we reached back to my parents' house. Most of us jumped into the pool to play

Marco Polo. The simple game of water tag had entertained us for more than thirty years. Dad fired up the grill. After dinner, Heather put on her snorkel gear and practiced.

A month later, from the fourth-floor balcony of a Florida Keys oceanside condo, Heather and I observed whitecaps frothing on inland waters, warning of a sea too rough for Heather's first trip to a coral reef. Out the door and down the stairs, wind gusts knocked over patio chairs, so we scratched any boating plans.

Near-shore shallow waters were calm for Heather to practice. Jim preferred staying dry and remained on-shore. Jamie, Tony, Heather, and I splashed in with our snorkel gear. Startled little crabs shot off in a puff of granules. A school of bonefish lazed along, rooting for small crustaceans. Undulating, a frightened octopus swam and wedged its soft body into a crevice, all but one tentacle hidden.

I'd long ceased to worry too much about sharks. Becoming somewhat rare, they were fast and elusive. Either a shark was hungry or not; and I might be its dinner or not. Overnight, fair weather calmed the ocean. Dad captained the twenty-one foot boat, sliding it along the glassy channel, pivoting gracefully through a maze of mangrove islands—intertwined, giant masses of leaves. An infinity of roots arched out of their stocky trunks a foot or so above the water's surface. Low tide would expose almost a meter more of the tapestry of living, interwoven wood.

The boat's propeller churned on, leaving behind a bubbly trail. The sun beat down from cerulean skies. Heather loved to ride on the open bow bench at the very front of boat, perched on her knees, letting the humid, salty wind blow her hair back.

Dad kept the red channel markers on our left, to navigate the deeper water, and not run aground on the flats.

"Can you see the next one?" Dad asked.

"A red one is straight ahead, with an osprey nest sprawled over."

We rounded the last island, and Dad slowed as he threaded his way through sandbars. A charter dive vessel approached from our port side.

"There's a funnel cloud out there!" the captain shouted.

"I see it," Dad replied, scanning the horizon.

"I said there's a funnel cloud!" the captain warned even more loudly.

"Thanks for the information," Dad answered, unconcerned. Storms moving through Key Largo's sunny skies travel fast and rarely send lightning. If you race toward a storm; they'll have moved on before you reach. The funnel cloud dropped farther, elongating two-thirds of the way down to meet the ocean, but the heavens beckoned and swallowed it back up. "Watch that location; the funnel might get spit out again," Dad cautioned.

"Waterspouts," I said, pointing to the north. Several spouts of spinning water and wind zoomed along the surface. They fizzled out quickly.

"Remember the eight dancing around Tavernier Key?" Dad asked.

"Those scared me, but with nowhere to run and hide, we relaxed and enjoyed the show."

Hot stillness vanished, and cool air blustered up whitecaps and whistled through the straps of the open boat's Bimini top. "Are you ready to get wet?" Dad asked.

Heavy sheets of rain reduced visibility to less than fifty feet. Dad slowed almost to a stop. The sunshade that covered the center console wasn't large enough to keep anyone dry. Heather and I huddled together to keep warm on the bow seat of the boat. We remained there to watch for darker-hued water that signifies patch reef. Towering mounds of coral rise from the bottom. Larger ones break through the surface or may be covered with only a few inches of water. Colliding with one might rip a hole in the hull, or the impact could jettison all of us. Dad veered south of the reef line until the bad weather dissipated.

Twenty minutes later, not a single cloud graced the horizon, and nary a boat. For a brief time, we owned the sea and the brilliant blue sky. Dad quickened our pace over waves that lifted the bow and dropped it with a slap, leaving light-weight Heather intermittently airborne. She loved it.

Locating a patch reef, Dad slowed, and shifted into idle. Jim gaffed the loop of the rope that attached to the mooring ball. He ran a dock line through the loop and knotted it to a bow cleat. "We are secure Fritz," Jim said. Dad shut off the engine.

Heather squirted jellyfish-repellant suntan lotion onto my back and rubbed it on, after which I slipped on a Lycra full bodysuit. For me, both were necessary barriers to seawater. Either the sea or I had changed. Without protection, contact with the ocean's stinging and nonstinging critters could blister most of my skin. With precautions, I could continue one of my most favorite pastimes.

Jamie shoved the large white cooler to the side and yanked on the metal pull ring of the center hatch to lift off its cover. She tossed out the stowed individual mesh bags of snorkel gear. I grabbed mine and jumped overboard.

"Feels like a sauna—come in and get warm. Gus is here. Don't kick him," I teased. Gus is our nickname for any large barracuda lurking underneath the boat. Lower jaw agape displaying razor-sharp peg-like teeth, about five-feet long, he looked right at me and cruised closer. His muscular, torpedo-shaped body was aluminum-colored and covered with fine scales. Two dark spots dotted his tail. An almost imperceptible movement sent him deeper into the shadow cast by the boat. There he lingered, waiting, in hopes that we were fishing, and he could snatch an easy dinner of hooked snapper.

Heather leapt in and treaded water. The plunge knocked off her mask. She spit onto its lens and rubbed saliva around as a coating to prevent fogging. In my mind, I gave thanks for the incredulous fruition of the dream. Heather could swim, and Heather could talk. Here she was, beside me, healthy forever daughter, snorkeling in the clear waters of John Pennekamp Coral Reef State Park. Little did I comprehend, it was still just the beginning of an unimaginable journey.

Tilting our heads underwater, we proceeded onward with slow kicks, dive flag in tow. Heather kept hold of my hand. A fat gag grouper hugged the bottom and disappeared under a ledge. Oodles of small transparent fry nestled into a soft brown finger coral tipped with purple. At the base of an enormous golden brain coral, a pair of angel fish hovered, their side fins flapping down to reveal a brilliant canary yellow.

We stopped swimming to float motionless, gazing downward, in hopes shyer creatures would venture out of hiding. Suspended above ancient corals and colorful fish, Heather and I held our breath and listened. Without noisy air rushing in and out of our snorkels, we almost ceased to exist. Incessant low clicking sounds of marine life engulfed us.

An approaching darkness alarmed me until I deciphered its looming mass—not a single creature, but millions of cave minnows, streaming in and conforming to coral heads as they fled from bar jacks that were herding them sheep-dog style. With a kick of our flippers, we descended and disappeared into the midst of the shiny minnows, letting them envelope us.

Up to the surface for some air, then a thrust of our flippers propelled us back toward the bottom. Twisting over onto our backs, we gazed upward, with the sole intent of observing the surreal art of exhaled air bubbles ascending to the surface where all coalesced, spreading into a flat glimmering, giant air globule with sunlight streaming through.

We swam over to my Dad who was trailing a green parrot fish and its incessant chomping bites of coral. Suddenly Heather gripped my fingers tighter. In her excitement, she popped up her head so she could speak aloud words that could be heard. "Fish! Look Mommy! Fish!" she exclaimed.

Below us, two majestic eagle rays glided in a pattern of wide and tilting ovals, seeming not to disturb a single molecule of water. A symmetrical gentle exertion of their dark wings, spanning wider than a tall man and swirled with almost contiguous circular markings of white, perpetuated their graceful dance. Each dragged behind a long skinny tail to counterbalance the weight of his stout body and head.

"Not often seen," I said in awe when Heather and I lifted our heads to converse.

"Excellent," Dad said.

Squinting at a rustic wooden sign that came into view, we swam closer to read. The reef marker warned, 'Keep Out, Research Only."

"Hey Dad!" I called him over.

"Whoops, how were we supposed to know?" he questioned.

Resuming our underwater exploration, I heard the rumble of a running boat motor and popped up to scan our surroundings and appraise any gonna-get-run-over danger. Dad and Heather heard it too, and the three of us treaded water.

The law-enforcement vessel approached, slowed, and stopped.

"Sorry, we couldn't read the signage from afar," Dad apologized.

"The issue is that you are supposed to remain within three hundred feet of your boat. Climb aboard, we'll give you a ride," the officer said.

His colleague objected. "They'll have to swim. It's against policy to take them on-deck,"

"I'll deal with you later," the marine patrol officer threatened. I don't know why he was so angry. Maybe he thought we'd been poaching fish and lobster.

Breaking all idle speed regulations, the officer raced off, neglecting mandatory perusal for surfacing divers. Suddenly, his boat bucked and reared like a stallion. Its prop had struck a coral head, slicing into it. The irate officer raised the motor to inspect for damage, then idled toward our boat. Jim had remained on-board to keep a watchful lookout on us. Jamie and Tony were sunning on deck.

"Swim slowly, better to arrive after that idiot has moved on." Dad suggested. Diving under. I saw where their prop gouged the brain coral. Pulverized fragments littered the bottom. On the surface, I watched as the officer tied his vessel up to our boat. Jim answered the man's terse questions and produced all requested paperwork. Somewhat satisfied, the officer retrieved his docking lines and sped off in his patrol boat.

At the condo that night, we grilled a chicken feast. Heather ran from aunt to uncle to cousin to grandma, hugging each of them before crawling onto my lap and throwing her arms around my neck. "Mommy, I was never worried. God told me I'd have a family," she said, speaking to both me and the group.

Suddenly sentimental, Dad asked, "What happens to the other voiceless children? What about that little boy with a trach? The one that got returned?"

"I don't know. Maybe another family reached out to him." Surprisingly, it had never entered my mind to give him a home. There is a limit to what one family can do.

She Can Swim!

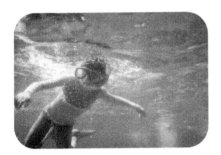 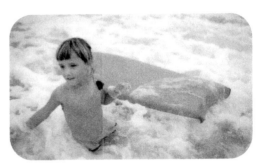

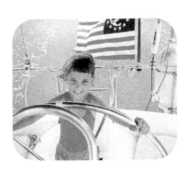 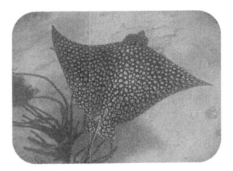

CHAPTER 22] TELL ME WHY

Life never returned to the simplicity of "before Heather." It changed from one of careful plans with expected outcomes to one of being surprised by inconceivable opportunities as we trod a new and brambly path, mostly with joyous hearts.

I tried to convince parents of children with tracheotomies to obtain a second opinion

from Dr. Maddern. Often the older surgeon who did the dilations would sway them against it. Most people had never heard of pediatric otolaryngology. There were only thirty-five in the world at the time. I did a lot of reading and peppered Dr. Maddern with on-going questions. Could what happened to Heather have been prevented? How to reach the scattered children with tracheotomies, so they could have a voice? And not just the literally voiceless children, what about the figuratively voiceless children in foster care?

Perhaps if I attended graduate school and earned a master's degree as a nurse-practitioner, I could have a greater positive impact.

Dr. Maddern suggested that I read the autobiography of Dr. Chevalier Jackson, the founder of bronchoscopy. The withering death of children who inhaled small toys or were stricken with diphtheria drove Dr. Chevalier Jackson to the crusade of developing safe airway examination in the late 1800s. He pioneered a way to glimpse into the lungs through his creation of surgical tools and development of specialized techniques. Prior to his innovative designs of a variety of bronchoscopes (instruments that pass from the mouth into the airways of the lungs), inhaling an object meant a quick or torturous death.

At the movie theater, Heather peered into the glass display case and pointed to a box of Sno-Caps. "Can I have a box of candy?" she asked.

"Yes," I answered. As the cashier handed over the chocolates and a sack of buttered popcorn, I felt a tap on my shoulder.

"Excuse me," the stranger said. "I noticed the scar on your child's neck. Your daughter looks so healthy. My granddaughter has a trach. She gets pneumonia a lot," she said.

"Heather used to be continually sick; now she seldom gets ill," I said, and proceeded to explain about the cartilage graft procedure. "Her voice sounds a bit breathy. One of her vocal cords doesn't move as it should. The resultant air leak muffles crisp pronunciation."

Ponytails bouncing with her enthusiasm, Heather chimed in. "Dr. Bruce fixed me." Heather lifted her shirt to show the scar along her lower ribs. "I can talk, and I can swim," she said with zest. "Last week, my granddad took me sailing."

"Lucky you; lucky grandfather," the woman said. "How old are you?" she asked.

"Four years old. Next year I'll play soccer like my sister and brother." Heather sparkled with anticipation.

"Please telephone my daughter and tell her about these newer options," she appealed, handing me the number, obviously wanting for her granddaughter all that Heather now enjoyed.

Every few months, Dr. Maddern had me speak with a mom nervous about her child's upcoming surgery and chat in a way that he couldn't. Not wanting to misinform, I proceeded to reread medical articles and search out new. Once I grasped the material, I would confirm my perceptions with Dr. Maddern. For example, I learned that a single intubation, even for a quick in-and-out look, can harm the trachea, especially in premature babies.

Most vulnerable to abrasive damage is where a breathing tube's far tip rests in the airway at the cricoid cartilage. The cricoid differs from other supporting tracheal cartilagine rings. It is the only one that forms a complete circle; the others are an open C-shape. Devoid of an anatomical shape that can give or expand, any injury to the cricoid can result in obstructive scarring; as happened to Heather.

Fortuitously, Heather and I continued to cross paths with children who breathed through tracheotomies. Chance introductions occurred at school, the grocery store, speech therapy, and a myriad of other coincidences. Causes of a child's tracheal scarring varied and included smoke inhalation during a house fire, facial anomalies, congenital airway defects, abnormal growths, or scarring from intubation for surgery or premature birth.

Always an opportunity arose for me to relay Heather's story to the tracheotomy child's parents. Ultimately each of those happenstance encounters led to successful reparative surgery by Dr. Maddern, followed by tracheotomy tube removal.

Jim had given my mom the go-ahead for the long ago promised dog.

"Grandy's on the phone and has something exciting to ask," Jamie said, beckoning me to hurry.

"I found an in-home breeder of Scottish Terriers near Orlando," Mom said. "She spoils the mamma dog and puppies. They have free range in a cordoned-off section of the kitchen. Only one female pup remains unsold. She has a thick, wiry coat, alert ears, and an affectionate disposition."

"Sounds terrific!" I said, and put Tony on the phone.

"Grandy, we're getting a girl dog?" Tony asked.

"Yes, in three weeks, you'll have your pup. How about naming her Meagan?" Mom suggested.

"Maybe when Meagan is bigger, she can have puppies." Tony was already making plans.

All of us were steeped in eager anticipation when Mom waltzed in with the little bundle of fluffy, black fur. Meagan's fat little tummy almost dragged the ground as she waddled toward the kids, stopping to piddle.

Bold, confident Heather caught us off-guard when she reacted with sudden fear to approaching four paws and her little pink tongue, just like she'd done that morning at the beach. She scurried away and clambered up onto the couch and kept climbing until she was atop the backrest. Perched there, she scrunched up her face and wailed.

Puppy responded with similar distress, whimpering louder by the moment. A few days later, Heather and the pup became friends. Inquisitive and teething, the pup chewed up Heather's pink prescription eyeglasses.

A home-care company was hiring registered nurses to care for very ill or ventilator-dependent children. After speaking with the director, I accepted a part-time position, and would work some of my off-days from labor and delivery.

My first assignment was caring for a little boy who'd been born with too few and non-working intestines. With the lack of working intestines, no food or water would move past his stomach, consequently he could not ingest and swallow any nourishment.

Toddling about, a medical pack was strapped to his back to carry a feeding solution that was pumped continuously through an access port into his venous blood. At the mom's insistence, a surgeon devised a way to let the child drink water without lethal sequelae. The caring surgeon created a stomach access, same as the gastrostomy button that Heather used to have, except it was used in reverse, as a drain. Any water that the boy sipped and swallowed would flow out of his stomach through the button to a collecting pouch belted to his abdomen. Without such a drain, water would stretch his stomach until it popped like a balloon.

Stoically, the boy's mother told me about her brush with child welfare. She'd experienced the heartache that the woman in foster-parent classes had warned about. Either well-meaning or malicious, a neighbor blamed the mother for the child's poor health and called the abuse hotline. Not understanding the child's illness, HRS seized the boy and moved him into medical foster care.

A guardian ad litem (GAL) helped her. Appointed by a judge, the GAL volunteer is a child advocate and conducts an independent investigation of a child abuse allegation. Meticulous documentation helped the mom prove that she was, in fact, an excellent parent. The state declared the abuse report unfounded and returned her child.

The state created the GAL program in an attempt to reduce harm caused by child-protection policy flaws. It's tricky to tease the truth out. In its zeal to protect a child from horrific situations, the court accepts anonymous abuse accusations as fact. No proof is required. False reports can trigger removal of children from their parents. Some innocent parents never get their children back. No one anticipated people calling in false hot line reports for their personal gain. The mother suggested that I become a GAL. I took the mother's suggestion and applied for training.

A GAL advocate is tasked with trying to ascertain the truth and representing the best interest of allegedly abused or neglected youth in courtroom proceedings. To better understand the health of a parent/child relationship—school, medical, and legal records are read; parents, family, neighbors, and teachers are interviewed. If youths have been placed in a foster-care home, the GAL volunteer is expected to make weekly visits to monitor their well-being.

Indeed, there are horrific cases of abuse, but often there is no abuse. Caseworkers, to justify their action of removing a child from a healthy home instead of admitting the error, are known to have fabricated damning allegations. No confirmation is required. The alleged witness might never be granted a chance to corroborate or refute, even if represented by a private attorney. The monster wheel keeps rolling cloaked in its guise of righteousness.

My next home-care nursing work assignment again exposed me to heartless bullying of the vulnerable. The child was a ten-month-old baby boy, who had a tracheotomy, rosy cheeks and a cherub's smile. A ventilator assisted him with his struggling breaths. He lived in a pleasant, beachside home with his teenage mother and grandma.

I was startled to hear the boy's doctor, who worked for the state, intimidating the young mom. For no reason, he threatened to have the oxygen-making machine removed. She responded with a flood of tears. I don't know why he proposed the preposterous thing. Fortunately the doctor didn't follow through with his evil statement. The family quietly endured any mistreatment that the man doled out, as they had no option of seeking medical care elsewhere.

On opening night of Holy Name of Jesus' annual fair, we were among the first to arrive. Jamie and Tony had sold enough advance tickets to win an unlimited-rides bracelet. Men of the parish spooned lacy balls of fried dough out of hot oil vats and dusted them with powdered sugar. Sticky fingered and eating funnel cakes, we walked toward the Gravitron. Heather dashed ahead and butted her way to the front. Jim caught up with her and retrieved her back to our place in line.

Inside the circular ride, we leaned back against its padded panels. Music blared, the automated doors closed, and the cylinder began to rotate, picking up speed. Centrifugal force pinned us to the wall, adhering us, as if stuck there by Velcro. Heather and Tony pivoted their bodies sideways, now horizontal to the floor. Jamie maneuvered to a diagonal. Then yuckiness. Jim threw up. After he tottered out of the machine, he hurled once more onto the grass. I murmured the unfortunate occurrence to the attendant.

Purposefully ignoring Jim's squeamishness, Heather dragged him onward to the Ferris wheel. Again she sprinted ahead to butt into the front of the line. Giving Jim a break, Jamie chased ahead and retrieved her little sister. Wisely, Jim stayed on level ground.

The Ferris wheel's rotation stopped when our cart was at the utmost top of the loop. For a quarter of an hour, we gently swayed there. "This is so fun!" Heather exclaimed. "I can see the ocean and river, and a really little Daddy." In high spirits, she waved down at him, standing below on the turf. He waved back. Next we rode the Zipper, with its spinning, twisting, and turn-you-upside-down thrills.

Heather and I veered off from the family group to take our assigned stint in the ring-toss booth. Carnival-style she touted chances to win stuffed animals, sizes ranging from small rabbits to enormous gorillas, while I handled the money. Once our replacement volunteers arrived, we ambled over to buy a cone of cotton candy and watch a few local dance troupes perform on stage. The fun didn't end with the weekend. Later in the month, the priest hosted a church dinner as his token of appreciation for all the volunteers.

Meeting Heather had vanquished the fallacy of self-reliance. On Sundays, we honored Father Walsh's almost decade-old request and attended mass. Afterward as a family, we served donuts in the church hall. Mass seemed to renew us through its dedicated time for prayer and meditation and communal sharing of God. Thoughtful gospels and homilies instilled a collective wisdom to live as best we can, one day at a time, and provided a contemplative foundation for improving our response to any future trouble. Joyful songs eased our fears and celebrated our blessings.

When Birgit, Dr. Maddern's medical secretary, called to confirm Heather's upcoming appointment, she had an intriguing request. We were to arrive two hours early so a photographer could snap photos of Heather for an informational brochure. "Everyone has been missing Heather. After her appointment, if it's agreeable, Dr. Maddern wants the two of you to join the office staff for lunch."

A couple of weeks later, Heather raced to hug Dr. Bruce.

"Look at you!" he said.

"I brought you a present. It is just like my doll," Heather said and handed him a Cabbage Patch doll, wearing an actual Shiley trach tube, inserted through a hole I'd whittled in the doll's hollow neck, with twill ties around and knotted.

"Thanks, Heather," Maddern said.

The photographer suggested that the finished medical brochure feature Heather on the cover, holding the special trach-doll. Throughout the photo shoot, Heather radiated happiness at hanging out with Dr. Bruce. She chatted amiably, becoming quiet and still only when instructed.

"She doing great," Dr. Maddern said to me.

"In one year, her vocabulary rocketed from zero to that of her four-year-old peers," I boasted. "Her voice is quiet though. She only exerts enough effort for us to understand. Others have difficulty, because she has little concern for distinct clarity."

To strengthen the muscles used for voice, Dr. Maddern recommended home practice guided by monthly appointments with the speech therapist in his clinic. Miss Judy specialized in teaching deaf children how to read lips and speak with their mouth. As such kids can not hear spoken words or those they utter, Judy used the tools of fingers feeling muscle movement and vibration as some of her methods to instruct.

I told Dr. Maddern about my frustration with medical politics. "Samantha's mom cancelled her daughter's appointment after talking with the older surgeon, the same one that Heather used to have. He spoke negatively about pediatric ear, nose, and throat surgeons," I said.

"But an idea sprouted when I was flipping through a magazine. If I can publish Heather's story as a feature article, I can bypass the good ole boys' resistance and reach out to children with tracheotomies all over the country, and educate doctors who are unfamiliar with pediatric ENT. That is, if I have permission to write about you? And if you'll proofread the medical part of what I write?"

"Go for it, Annie," Dr. Bruce encouraged. At his request, Heather and I went by the hospital room of a sick baby to answer his mother's questions and provide hope. In the near future, the baby would undergo the same surgical procedures that opened Heather's airway.

"I'm sorry; I can't help staring. Your daughter is healthy!" the woman said.

Equally moved, Heather drew closer to the crib. "I want to be Dr. Maddern. I'd get the baby's trach out, so he could talk," Heather said.

Driving home, we detoured through Gainesville. A stop at Shands Hospital, and a stroll to PICU to show off a thriving

Heather. We learned that good fortune had come to Alex, the boy with the trach whose potential parents had returned him. After residing in the PICU for more than three years, a medical student and his wife adopted the boy and moved out of state. No one knew whether he still had the trach.

CHAPTER 23]
GUARDIAN

I whispered to Heather that for the moment we were lost, somewhere in the scrub brush of Canaveral National Seashore.

"Don't alarm the foster kids," I said. I had taken them on an outing for my weekly GAL visit. I'd finished the training and accepted an assignment. We were all fatigued.

The young boy and girl had been emergency removed from their home. The judge formally appointed me as their guardian ad litem. I had been checking on them at their foster home for months. Close in age to Heather, who was then five years old, she usually tagged along on any outings.

As the afternoon waned, the path we were following hadn't led us back to the parking lot as I'd expected. Biding time to gather my bearings, we stopped and observed waterfowl preening their feathers at the edge of a pond. I surmised that if we could keep the afternoon sun warming our backs, we'd walk east and not in circles.

"Keep it fun. Suggest a butterfly hunt, okay?" I quietly asked Heather.

"Let's search for an orange monarch, or a beautiful blue butterfly. I can fly like one. Come along." Heather pantomimed the delicate insect's motions and pretended to flit across some flowers. The two kids mimicked her. They enjoyed skipping down the trail, pausing to look over blossoms for quavering wings or stooping to overturn rocks. Imagination sustained the tired ones until around a bend, I located the parking lot and the van.

I kept all of the GAL course examples in mind as I reviewed the children's records and talked with people who knew the family. The instructor stressed great awareness and skepticism when conducting an independent investigation. It was important to understand how the system worked because of the many people I'd met and the stories they'd told, some good, some bad. The course instructor said false hotline calls might spring from spiteful ex-spouses, well-meaning acquaintances, ignorant meddlers, and errant professionals.

System flaws can make it impossible for a falsely accused parent or one needing remediation to accomplish what the state requires. Caseworkers might never provide parents notice of mandatory court appearances, perhaps due to carelessness, ignorance, or deliberate personal agenda. If parents do not know to attend, their opportunity to speak is lost. If a judge grants a new chance, a caseworker may have already coerced parents to remain silent, by threatening to cancel upcoming visits with their baby or child if they talk to the judge.

Rules were tightened up with the intention of children not languishing in foster care for numerous years. Parents have a case plan of tasks to accomplish. Some parents lack transportation, and so can be improbable. They might not have money to pay for mandatory parenting courses or random drug testing. Attending court and fulfilling case plan requirements might cause a parent to miss too much work, and subsequently get laid off. Holding a job is often requisite to regain custody of your children.

A caseworker may withhold the list of mandatory tasks until three months after a child's removal. The tasks may take six months to accomplish; and the state expects them done within six months.

Yet the timer began ticking on day one, not on distribution day ninety. Failure is guaranteed. The mother and father will have their parental rights permanently terminated. Their former children will remain in foster care, until categorized as adoptable and selected by new parents.

Though at first hesitant, actually at first frightened, what if they were really monster parents? I'd come to trust the parents-under-scrutiny enough to visit with them periodically. I helped them figure out which bus routes would get them to required classes. I gave the mother rides when transportation was not available. When I had completed my report, the judge reviewed the findings of my independent investigation and arranged a confidential hearing in his private chambers.

His Honor commenced the proceedings with an opening story of coincidence. For breakfast, he'd stopped at a small diner. "Who happened to sit at the next table, but these parents in question. I observed their actions, unbeknownst to them or to me that I would shortly thereafter render a decision about their children." He emphasized an important point. "One parent can have problems; only one parent has to be stable," he specified.

Turning to me, he said he had a few questions, with strict guidelines on how I was to respond. "Answer 'yes' or 'no;' no elaboration. Would you have the children returned home?" asked the judge.

"Yes," I answered.

"Today?" he asked.

"Yes," I said, without hesitation.

That I was surprised at his next question to me is a vast understatement. He prefaced his request by saying he had a concern, no one knew whether one or both parents might drive drunk. "Until the next hearing and it gets sorted out, would you drive the children to Busy Bear Day Care? It will be for only one week."

"Yes," I replied.

The children were taken out of foster care and returned home to their parents that afternoon. Neither parent was allowed to drive with their children in the vehicle.

The day-care itself was part of the on-going investigation. Teachers were tasked with observing the children and reporting any injuries or strangeness to the court.

Despite the judge's assurances, the hearing was repetitively postponed and my one-week commitment stretched out to six. Translated, that means I drove a total of sixty morning pick-ups and evening drop-offs. Heather always accompanied me, as she was too young for public school. During the commute, we conversed with the children.

At each collecting and depositing of children, she and I went inside the trailer and chit-chatted with sober parents. Through such frequent and sequential contact, I accumulated first-hand glimpses into their parenting and homemaking; gaining even greater confidence in my original findings.

For the next hearing, we again gathered in the judge's private chambers. The judge declared the hotline allegations unfounded. "Poverty is not a reason for removal of children. There's been no abuse or neglect," he stated his decision with finality. He reinstated the parents' right to drive with their children in the car. He stipulated that the parents participate in certain beneficial social classes.

For many years afterward, the family invited us over to their home during the Christmas holidays. We'd exchange small gifts. Jim would assist them with computer enhancements. Heather enjoyed renewing her friendship with the young boy and girl. The father always expressed gratitude prior to our leaving. "Each night the children and I get on our knees and thank God for your intervention. We pray for blessings for you and your family."

As rewarding as the experience was, I never took on another GAL assignment. Mostly because my idea of publishing a magazine feature about Heather and the miracles wrought by pediatric otolaryngologists became my foremost priority.

To succeed required two years of concentrated effort. Obsessed with what seemed an ordained quest, I pored over books on writing into the wee hours trying to learn the craft. In the early stages, I travelled to Gainesville on weekends so I could toil at the creative process with Celeste sitting beside me, tossing words, critiquing, and dreaming. She typed my handwritten pages until I learned the skill. Jim gifted me with our first computer to streamline the process and make the infinite revisions easier.

I condensed the story of Heather up-to-that-point into a few pages. After tossing a mountain of drafts into the trash, I began pitching the idea to major magazines via a query letter. Nearing my hundredth rejection, I attended my first Space Coast Writers' Conference. At the sign-in table, I picked up a succinct flyer advertising the editorial services of Julia Lee Dulfer.

As she worked, she would visualize the pictures that the written words portrayed or how they failed to do so, and the music of the stringing of those words. Twice a month, I began meeting with fellow writers in her home. She would read a member's piece and explain her thought process, as she strengthened the grammar and structure and taught us the art of writing. Never did she change the style, nor do the writer's thinking. The quality of the end result was always limited by the author's persistence, skill, rewriting, and polish.

One month later, after a single edit by Julia Lee, the manuscript was accepted by *Woman's Day*. It appeared in the May 18, 1993 issue as "The Child No One Wanted," and was later reprinted in England's *Woman* and Germany's *Bildwoche*.

Over the summer, Heather's speed on the soccer field earned her the nickname, "Dynamo." In September, six-year-old Heather began kindergarten. The first day of school, she wore a plaid skirt, a cotton shirt decorated with a Scotty-dog appliqué, and sturdy tortoise-shell glasses perched on her nose. Her bangs fell to a smidgeon above her eyebrows.

Heather knelt down to pet her beloved dog, Meagan. She and Tony shrugged on their backpacks. We took photographs, using the coquina rock out-front as the stage. Heather's face shone with strong, happy confidence as she pedaled her yellow bicycle alongside her brother and me toward the neighborhood elementary school.

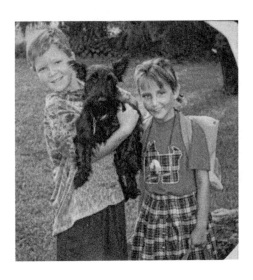

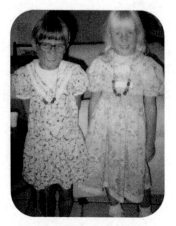

Heather & Robyn

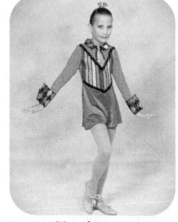

Tap dancer

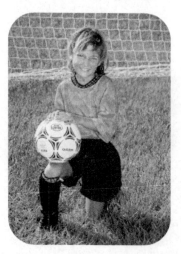

Dynamo

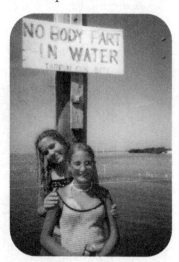

Florida Keys

Despite those early predictions of severe disability, she did the curriculum and was like the other kids in her class except for health information posted in the clinic on her behalf. Her handwriting was shaky. Her speech still sounded soft as she preferred to move her lips the minimum possible, and a trifle breathy due to a unilateral partial vocal-cord paralysis. No teachers or children ever made derogatory comments about her voice. Most had first met Heather when she had her tracheotomy and could not speak at all.

Cousins Bryan and Daniel came over for the afternoon of a school holiday. Using their imagination, the troop of cousins shoveled a sandy spot in the backyard near the tangerine tree. "Only Aunt Ann would let us dig for treasure like this," Bryan piped up. In the wide pit, he stood chest-deep. Dripping sweat, the kids changed into their bathing suits. Cooling off in our circular aboveground pool, they all swam in the same direction along the outer edge to create a whirlpool effect. Hopping out, they shoveled in spurts, filling in the deep hole.

After showers, we watched the movie, *Tarzan*. Heather wasn't good at sitting still. She darted about into this and that and over to Meagan, who had her paws on the windowsill, barking excitedly for two reasons. Heather investigated the ruckus. A lizard was rhythmically puffing out its ruby-red throat, and Jim was pulling into the driveway.

Vibrant Heather burst out the front door to greet her dad, as she did each evening, reaching him as he stepped from the car. She had something extra special to announce. "Daddy! Daddy! Daddy! Guess what? I'm going to be on TV with Dr. Bruce."

"Yippee!" Jim exclaimed. Acting on a sudden impulse, he stepped onto the lawn and flipped into a celebratory handstand, legs straightening toward the sky. His undershirt shimmied down his upside-down chest, baring his flat abdomen. I crept over and tickled his belly. With a happy laugh, he tumbled onto the grass. I told him how reporters for WJXT, Channel 4 evening news in Jacksonville, wanted to run a segment featuring Heather's surgical success. One of them had read the story in *Woman's Day*.

Dr. Bruce called to set a date for the filming at his office. "Barbara and I would like you and Heather to stay with us. Come on, Annie, you'll have your own room and bathroom," he insisted. We did, and Heather slept in with their youngest child, Alexis.

Broadcast day, WJXT's television signal wouldn't reach Indialantic, but Gainesville could receive it. Coverage began early morning with the news team promoting viewership throughout the day with glowing preview clips of "a remarkable adoption story." Ecstatic about the quality of previews and the feature, Mark and Celeste phoned us details and mailed a video copy.

The filmmakers captured the beauty and spirit of our serendipitous Heather. Reporter Tom Willis introduced the story with these opening remarks: "You need a big heart, loads of patience, and a real drive to help an ill child get a good start in life." The camera scanned the scenic St. Johns River. It showed me catching Heather midair as she jumped off a tree branch. She looked cute and charismatic in her blue-and-white dress and hair in two ponytails. Cameras zoomed in on her singing "Itsy Bitsy Spider," using dramatic hand motions for "washed the spider out."

"Ann says Dr. Maddern's the reason her little girl can sing songs and tell stories today," reporter Mary Baer said. "The doctor himself fights back tears when he thinks about this courageous little girl."

"It's a very nice outcome to a potentially sad, sad story. That's why we're in the business of doing these kinds of surgeries—to have results like this," Dr. Maddern answered.

"The Gigantis encourage other families to take the risk and adopt special-needs kids. That's why Ann wrote her marvelous article," Mary Baer said. The camera zoomed in on Heather and me sitting on a park bench. Superimposed like a shadow, the pages of the *Woman's Day* article scrolled along, as I read its words to her.

"The power of love," Deb Gianoulis declared emphatically in closing.

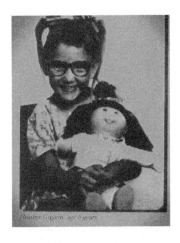

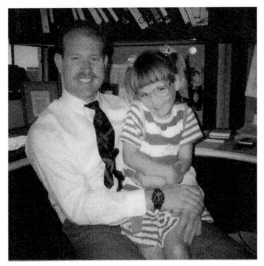

Dr. Bruce Maddern & Heather, after filming for WJXT news

A boon resulted. The Academy of Otolaryngology's administrator offered me a journalist's pass—unlimited access to all events at their national meeting in Minneapolis, if I provided my own transportation and lodging.

On arrival to the largest of the Twin Cities, I checked into my room at the conference's primary hotel. Changing into a one-piece swimsuit, I burned off the novelty of traveling by myself by swimming laps in the heated pool. In the elevator, wet hair wrapped in a towel and sweat pants on, I conversed with an older couple who were attending the convention. The husband stood with the aid of crutches strapped to his forearms. He spoke about nothing specific and asked a few questions about Florida's weather.

For the next morning's opening meetings, I wore a feminine blouse and dark pants and jacket to blend in with the conservative gathering. Executive vice-president, Dr. Jerome Goldstein, warmly welcomed me and issued the all-inclusive admission badge.

The business assembly was about to commence. I looked out over a collage of gray and balding heads of the predominately male Caucasian crowd. The attendants forbade my entrance into the room, until I showed them the pass. I walked toward the speaker's podium. About a third of the way from the front, I sidestepped down an empty row to a seat in the middle.

Ten minutes later, the man whom I had met in the elevator, who had the arm crutches, laboriously made his way to the seat next to mine. He introduced himself, Dr. Greg Steadman. During a break, I told him about Heather and my foray into writing. He suggested that I introduce myself to Dr. Lauren Holinger. The surgeon's father, Dr. Paul Holinger, had brought otolaryngology to the United States from Switzerland. His aunt Alice had known Dr. Chevalier Jackson and was great friends with his son.

Wandering around the exhibits, I met Dr. Maddern's mentor, Dr. Sylvan Stool. Intelligent and humble, the surgeon completed two formal residencies, first as a pediatrician, then as an otolaryngologist. A gracious man, he welcomed my questions with kindness and joviality. Before the 1970s, almost all premature babies who weighed less than three pounds, would die. Survival depended on "someone hand-squeezing a breathing bag to keep oxygen flowing. A tiny baby could be kept alive, maybe for twenty-four hours at the most. Being dependent on human energy, you couldn't keep going—you ran out of people," he said.

"Before electrically powered breathing machines, whole groups of people succumbed—babies, children, and adults. The initial ventilators pumped in a prescribed volume that didn't adjust to changing resistance, so they often damaged and popped the delicate tissue of a baby's lungs.

"Not before they developed a pressure-controlled ventilator, a machine that could make a primitive decision to build to a certain pressure, stop and release that pressure, and be set to cycle a fixed number of times per minute could premature babies be kept alive until their lungs matured." He credited the space program for developing the breakthrough technology, made possible through its development of pressure transducers, smaller motors, and improved ways for monitoring the body's oxygen and carbon dioxide levels.

"The first success came in 1968," Dr. Stool said. "A premature infant was ventilated for about nine months. Just today before coming here I looked at a baby picture of him showing his tracheotomy. At the time I estimated the cost of his hospitalization at dollars per inch of the chart's thickness—$250,000, which seemed astronomical….That he did survive intact and beautiful was a powerful stimulus for other neonatal units to succeed at repeatedly reproducing the same result. Perhaps it made him one of the most expensive babies in the world. Two or three years ago he graduated from college."

In 1968, he immediately recognized the dangers created by the success. "Oh what had we done?" He'd pondered the magnitude of the resultant miracles, tragedies, and moral dilemmas. If a ventilator can prolong a baby's life that would have ended in death, when is it not appropriate?

Ending the conversation, I walked on to Dr. Lauren Holinger's course on foreign body aspiration. "A whole platoon—toy soldiers, navy ships, army helicopters, coins, jewelry, and nuts—I've removed them all from children's lungs," he said. Afterward I told him about amazing Heather. Dr. Holinger wrote a letter of introduction to his Aunt Alice.

CHAPTER 24]
CHEVALIER JACKSON

Yikes, the bunny dug out! Heather shouted and sprinted after him. As a lanky eight-year-old, she was in charge of feeding Fluffy, the pet rabbit. Fearing our two dogs would hunt him as prey, his outdoor hutch was kept inside a fenced run that we periodically dragged to a fresh spot of grass.

Heather kept up the chase, but Fluffy scampered out-of-reach under the canoe. The dogs flushed him out. Rabbit hopped behind some colorful croton bushes. Surprising us all, the dogs seemed to regard bunny as an inedible peer. The trio continued their new game: find your friend and scamper. When Fluffy had enough of tag, he squirmed back under the fenced run and hopped into his hutch. The pets continued to play most days.

Heather carried herself in a slightly clumsy way. No matter the amount of practice for dance class, she hadn't limbered up enough to ease into a backbend. At school, her teachers worried about her reading comprehension and handwriting skills. They didn't push. Heather always strived and gave her best efforts.

About twice a month, all three of my kids or just Heather, would go with me on my day off to visit the various children that I cared for in their homes. It gave mine an awareness, and Heather bestowed hope. Heather read *The Cat in the Hat* to the sickly siblings. Observant Heather tuned in, easily befriending them. She seemed blind to the torturous bodies and easily perceived their sweet essence.

My agency had sent me to the house of an older couple, Ed and Nancy Bristol (Saint Ed and Saint Nancy), who are the most generous couple that I have ever met. Motivated by compassion, they'd taken into their home five bed-ridden or wheelchair-bound children. One had severe autism; most had CP (cerebral palsy). None walked. None could sit without tethers.

A chalkboard, almost the size of an entire living-room wall, harbored the litany of appointments and therapies.

This family, too, had experienced the sting of HRS. An unwitting caseworker removed the kids. Nancy and Ed somehow got them back. To avoid a recurrence and block routine visits from HRS to their home, they turned down the state's offer of monthly monetary subsidies, relying instead on private donations.

Personal grief is what ignited Nancy's compassion. As a young adult, she had begged to have her younger sister reside with her. Instead their mother placed the child, who suffered from cerebral palsy, into an institution. None of the facility's staff assisted the girl with eating, and she starved to death.

Nancy showed me a photograph of teenager Jeff's latest bronchoscopy. Bumpy red scarring bubbled up at the carina, the place where the trachea splits into the right and left bronchi. It was the same spot that a suction catheter hits when inserted deep until meeting resistance.

"Dad and I used to suction you," I said, as I showed the picture to Heather. "That sore spot in Jeff's lungs is called a granuloma, and is caused by suctioning." I explained how Jim and I were taught to insert a catheter through the trach, sliding it along her delicate airway tissues to that same deep spot; but it seemed to hurt her, so we began stopping way short.

I offered no suggestions on suctioning technique for Jeff; I did not know enough. His situation seemed different. He did not even have a tracheotomy tube, just cerebral palsy.

On our way home from the Bristols, Heather and I stopped at 7-Eleven for a triple-flavor mix Slurpee. As we pulled in to the driveway, Heather clambered out of the van, eager to speak with her dad about her day at school. "For show-and-tell, I shared how Tony saved the turtle from getting squished by cars. They thought it was cool. Specially how it got scared when Tony picked it up off the road, and it peed like a gushing fire hydrant. And I told the class that Tony is a good soccer goalie. In poster club, I drew my brother diving and blocking a ball from scoring into the net."

"Awesome," Jim said.

Heavy rains loomed over the river, so Heather's coach called off soccer practice. On a whim, Jim proposed shopping for a new bike.

"Yes! Daddy, you're the best!" Heather whirled around with eager anticipation. Jamie went with them to critique the options. I chose to stay home and relax. In everyday life, Heather romped about, easy to please; but shopping with me always had her switching gears. She wanted it all, and her impatience with any limitation led to melt-downs and tears. Not so with Jim; she kept the charm on.

They selected a pink girl's bike with training wheels that had to be shipped from the warehouse. On delivery day, Heather wrote in her school journal, "I'm getting a new bike today. It's coming in a box. I already know what my bike looks like because I went to the store and pikt one out that I wanted but they didn't have one to give me. My new bike will be shinny and gliterley. I have scoccer today."

Amazing. After Dr. Lawrence Holinger penned the letter to his Aunt Alice, she phoned and invited me to visit in Pennsylvania. Heather wished that she could come along. Next time, I promised.

I flew in a day early to downtown Philadelphia so I could tour the Mutter Museum. I stared, mesmerized at the displays. They'd neatly categorized two-thousand foreign bodies that Dr. Jackson had personally removed from a patient's lungs, esophagus, or stomach. Also on display was an extensive collection of medical devices that Chevalier Jackson had developed.

Many of the patients who sought treatment from Dr. Jackson were starving, emaciated children. Each had ingested household lye from unlabeled containers thinking it was sugar. The caustic substance burnt the throat and esophagus, creating strictures that impeded swallowing. Such happenings reinforced Dr. Jackson's belief that "The work of physicians in prevention equals their work in curing disease." For twenty-five years, he lobbied the government to require that packages of lye substances be labelled in large letters: POISON. Success came in 1927, when President Coolidge signed the Federal Caustic Act.

I rang Alice Finkh's doorbell. The elderly woman was stooped and wore a soft dress, her smile and demeanor enchanting. We sat in upholstered wing chairs. She reminisced about her brother Paul and the spectacular life-saving foreign body cases. "Not for meanness, Paul refused when a child asked to have back the toy that he'd just plucked from the small child's delicate lungs. He didn't want the play thing to endanger the child, again."

Alice and her late husband were fortunate to have dined with Chevalier Jackson, Sr. They did so on four occasions, rare occurrences as he preferred working or resting with his family. "He usually went to bed early, placing a beverage and a sandwich wrapped in wax paper onto his bedside table. At 4:00 or 5:00 a.m., he'd eat the waiting snack for breakfast and commence his voluminous medical writing."

Dr. Charles Norris, who took over the endoscopy (airway or esophageal examination) clinic, joined us for tea. "Dr. Jackson removed objects from the lungs with almost complete success. If a modification or a newly designed instrument was needed to access and remove a foreign body, Jackson would jog over to Pilling & Son Company. The instrument-maker would take his sketches and manufacture the new tool overnight so as to be available for Dr. Jackson's use in endoscopy the next day. Have you seen the x-ray of the baby who had four open safety-pins lodged in his esophagus?"

"Yes, in his autobiography, he called them 'danger-pins'!"

Their busy endoscopy clinic was open three mornings a week, with cases scheduled at ten-minute intervals. Foreign bodies were perhaps fifteen percent of the schedule. To expedite things, while one patient was in the operating room, the next patient had a numbing surface anesthesia sprayed over the throat and down the windpipe. The person would remain breathing on his own. No going to sleep as there was not room in the trachea for both an examining bronchoscope and a ventilating tube.

"One unforeseen consequence was very difficult for Dr. Jackson," Dr. Norris said. "It was that he himself could use his instruments with reasonable safety, but in other doctor's hands, the tools became instruments of death. Thinking the introduction of a bronchoscope or esophagoscope simple, the unpracticed surgeon often perforated the lung or esophagus; and the patient would die."

The misfortune of numerous deaths made Dr. Chevalier Jackson, Sr. feel that he should never have crafted the tools. To curb the tragedies, he began offering courses for physicians to develop the necessary hands-on skills to perform safe bronchoscopy and esophagoscopy.

The following day, Alice Finkh and I dined at one of her favorite restaurants. Afterward we drove to Chevalier Jackson's homestead, Old Sunrise Mills. He'd purchased the historic property in the early 1900s. An actual mill, and one of only a few that could process wood and grain. It had supplied both to the troops wintering at Valley Forge during the Revolutionary War.

Envisioning the past came easily, for the land was unchanged from when the brilliant doctor lived there. In awe of all he accomplished, we peeked into the old tool house, which is where Jackson had his workshop and designed his instruments. While touring his extensive property we met his great-granddaughter, Susan Ruby. She showed us some of his original bronchoscopes. At the end of my visit, Alice Finkh gave me a print of one of the oil canvases that Chevalier Jackson painted of his home. I thanked her for a most extraordinary week.

Later that year, my family walked the grounds of Sunrise Mills with me. The children and I had accompanied Jim on a business trip to Philadelphia. Listening to the cascading water and inhaling the fragrance of pines, Heather scampered around like an inquisitive squirrel. "See that little boat resting against the stone house? Dr. Chevalier Jackson would paddle it to the far edge of the millpond so he could write undisturbed. His pioneering work paved the way for Dr. Maddern to give you a voice," I said to Heather.

Back at the hotel, Heather snuggled under her comforter, all ready for sleep. "I hope it snows," she said. Rising early, she peeked through a break in the curtains, and drew them open. "Daddy look! I knew it would happen," she said, waking him by tugging at his pajama sleeve. Together they gazed at the winter wonderland.

Eager for the children to experience their first snow, warm jackets on, we moseyed outside. Jim, Jamie, Tony, and Heather flopped backward onto the powdery snow and moved their arms and legs as in jumping jacks before springing up. Jamie snapped pictures of the snow-angel imprints and their snow-flake-dusted human counterparts. Lacking sleds, we scavenged for cardboard boxes, flattened them, and rode the temporary toboggans down nearby snow-covered hills.

Back in Florida and at work caring for the youngest child at the Bristols', sickly since birth. She had a tracheotomy. Her hospital bed was in the family room. On the other side, in another hospital bed, was the teenager, Jeff. His body's severe spasticity twisted him, rendering him barely able to move and unable to talk. Nancy believed he had a superior mind imprisoned in his uncooperative body.

Jeff's body language reacted as he watched his favorite movie, *My Left Foot*, a true story of a youth afflicted with cerebral palsy. In the movie, the boy's only mobile body part was his left foot. Impoverished, his healthy siblings accomplished their schoolwork by scratching their lessons on the floor with chalk, while the boy lay on the floor nearby. To their amazement, the boy grabbed a chunk of chalk with his good toes and began scrawling words.

The movie spawned hope that we might procure for Jeff an adaptive computer designed so as to accommodate his limited ability to operate it, opening for him the possibility of boundless communication.

Nancy was troubled because Jeff had been losing weight even though she had increased the quantity and caloric value of his tube feedings. Something clicked in my thoughts about weight loss caused by difficulty in breathing. His tongue hardly ever retrieved inside his mouth; mainly it jutted out over his lower lip and rested on his very small, recessed chin.

"Okay if I listen with a stethoscope?" I asked. As his chest moved, I heard air rushing in and out of his lungs until dramatically the sounds ceased, though his chest heaved with increasing effort. He contorted his body in paroxysms until he swung his rigid arms and repositioned himself to where his airway reopened. I heard the resumption and soft rustling of moving breath.

"I know the problem," I stated. "Intermittently he completely obstructs his airway."

Jeff's beaming gratitude for my sudden recognition of his stressful predicament spread into a happy guffaw that enveloped his whole body, racking him with more spasticity.

"Ann figured it out, Ann figured it out," his mom chanted. Nancy and I danced a swing for Jeff's amusement, and the giddy laughter of relief consumed him even more. My little-girl patient, whose intellectual and physical selves were severely crippled, joined in the foolery with a smile and animated eyes.

I phoned Dr. Maddern to discuss Jeff's situation. "Would you examine him?" I asked.

"Today, if you think he needs hospitalization," Dr. Maddern replied

"He does," I said.

"Let Birgit know once he's on the way. We'll make all arrangements for his admission to pediatrics," he said.

Nancy called Children's Medical Services (CMS) for transportation to Wolfson Children's Hospital in Jacksonville. They hesitated and said they would get back to her, so she bypassed them and directly contacted a Medicaid-accepting transporter. A few hours later CMS replied that providing transport was impossible.

"Oh really," Nancy replied, and proudly reported the opposite. Jeff had been picked up by a medical van and was almost to his destination.

Dr. Maddern examined Jeff and determined that the base of Jeff's tongue obstructed his airway severely. He needed a tracheotomy. Down the road it might become feasible to do a fancier tongue modification procedure and eliminate his need for a trach.

Jeff's surgery went fine. Nancy or Ed had to complete tracheotomy-care training. Their van was in poor shape, so Ed and I drove together in my station wagon.

"Did you ever think you'd care for handicapped kids at age seventy-two?" I asked Ed.

"Never crossed my mind that I'd do so at any age," Ed replied.

Stopped at a gas station, as I selected the fuel grade to fill the tank, an attendant offered to check the oil. He opened the hood. I didn't pay attention to what he was doing.

"Lady, your vehicle's going to blow up if you go any farther," he said.

Too dramatic, I'd heard that line before, directed to a timid college friend. Figuring Ed and I looked like the ultimate suckers, we took our chances and kept on driving.

Congenial Barbara Maddern offered hospitality, but Ed preferred to lodge at the Ronald McDonald house. I accepted an overnight stay in the Madderns' home. Ed completed his training. The results were fabulous. Jeff was no longer terrorized by impending suffocation. After returning from the hospital, he could breathe effortlessly through the tracheotomy. Amazing results followed. Jeff gained twenty pounds in the first month.

CHAPTER 25]
GAINING
KNOWLEDGE

At home, our dog was pregnant. Heather sat close to Meagan, peering down at the tummy bulging with growing puppies.

Heather's bangs covered the upper edge of her eyebrows, and her glasses slid down her nose. "Mom, come feel the kicking. Lots of squirmy, rolling movements; how many do you think she'll have?" she asked. Restless, mamma dog got up and moseyed over to sniff under the dining table and proceeded to paw at the hallway throw rug.

"Maybe it's whelping time," Jim said. To serve as a birthing box, he positioned a plastic kiddie pool in the middle of the living room and lined it with newspapers and old towels. Heather dangled a meatball in front of our dog's nose and coaxed her to jump in. Waiting for any confirmatory telltale signs, we sat around and watched television. After a couple of hours, everyone except Heather and me went to bed.

Eventually I too grew tired and retreated to slumber land. Heather refused to sleep and insisted on tending to her furry friend. Her watchful eyes saved a new life.

"Mom! Mom! Come quick," she pleaded, waking me. "Meagan pulled her back paw up, scratching. I saw tiny puppy feet, but its tail is stuck." Arriving backward into this world, hind legs out. Halting the whole process, its little stub of a tail poked through the thin, stretched tissue surrounding the birth canal. I freed the stub, and the mamma's contracting muscles squeezed out her pup.

Meagan dawdled, so I peeled off the amniotic sac from the newly born's nostrils, head, and body. The wet, furry wee one sagged limply and made no effort to breathe. Remembering Celeste's story of resuscitating a newborn kitten, I gently puffed air into the pup's little nostrils. After the assisted start, the pup continued breathing.

"Good job, Heather," I said. Breech births are risky because the after-following larger head often gets stuck. We wakened Jim, Jamie, and Tony. All hurried back. Heather massaged our beloved pet. Five additional puppies were born. Each emerged head first. Each time, mamma dog dawdled, and I had to peel off the translucent birth sac. Meagan licked the wet fur dry, simultaneously stimulating each pup's stretch for air. Joyous over the births, Heather and I curled up on the nearby floor with a blanket and went to sleep. The others straggled back to their beds.

In a few weeks, the fat little pups could scramble out of the plastic pool. We moved them to a higher-walled enclosure, the tile tub of the hallway bathroom. Growing bigger, they could sprawl their front paws and noses over the upper edge, but not get out. Coal black eyes peered at us longingly. Begging intensified to incessant barking. For quiet, we rewarded their persistence by removing them to roam freely on the back porch.

Cousins Bryan and Daniel came over to play with the puppies.

"Aunt Ann, can I have the fattest boy?" Daniel asked hopefully.

"Sure, but call your parents."

"Mom agreed, though she prefers a girl. How about the timid one?" He gathered her up, and she clung to him like a koala hugging a tree branch.

"Good choice, maybe name her something Scottish?"

"Loch Ness Monster," Daniel replied.

"How about Vanessa, Queen of Loch, but call her Nessie?"

Spirited Nessie travelled home with Daniel as soon as she reached two months old. Ears and tail up, she cavorted about in a style befitting her royal name. Daniel carried Nessie everywhere, pampering her and snuggling her close. Yet the match lasted only a few days. My sister's husband disliked the breed. He wanted the family dog to be a Boykin, same as his childhood dog, and delivered an edict. "The puppy goes."

Nessie boomeranged to Jim and me, boosting our family to include two dogs, a guinea pig, a cockatiel, three rabbits, two daughters, and one son.

Heather was faring pretty well in school, but often flunked standardized testing. She was having increasing trouble with ear infections. She coughed almost every day. An x-ray showed her lungs to be quite scarred, with areas of collapse and areas of hyperinflation. Unfortunately, our older daughter, Jamie, also seemed prone to bronchitis and sometimes flared up with hard breathing, so much so that we had to rent a wheelchair to push her along at our last outing to an Orlando theme park.

My compulsion to discover how Heather's medical problems might have been prevented and to learn more, led me to apply to the University of Central Florida's new degree offering. I received a letter of acceptance into the first class of students studying their nurse-practitioner curriculum. Graduation would be my entrance ticket to a greater vantage point from which to make a difference.

That photo of Jeff's airway settled my choice of topics for the required graduate-school research paper, which I titled "Airway

Suction, Not So Simple." I read more than three hundred research articles. Adverse effects of suctioning include: irregular heart rhythms, infection, granulomas, hypoxia, stripped mucosa, increased intracranial pressure with bleeding, and lung puncture, deflation, and collapse.

Bruce Maddern agreed to lead my advisory committee and confirmed many suspicions. Inspecting many tracheas with the laryngoscope, he often found suction-abrasion damage at the carina and elsewhere.

My writing moved forward, too. Over the phone, I pitched an idea for an article about Heather's airway reconstructive surgery to the editor at *MCN: The American Journal of Maternal/Child Nursing*. Lucky again, she gave the go-ahead to write "Lifesaving Tubes, Lifetime Scars?"

Preferring to have first-hand knowledge of the operation, I asked Dr. Maddern to secure permission for me to observe him perform a laryngotracheoplasty at Wolfson Children's Hospital. I was agog at how life had brought me to that particular point. *Pinch my arm and wake me up*, I thought as I changed into scrubs, mask, bouffant hair cap, and shoe covers in the surgical dressing room.

Marveling at the refined expertise of Dr. Maddern and his team, I watched as he incised the airway of a three-year-old foster child, like Heather had once been. I scribbled careful notes about each detail of the surgery. Later, referring to the meticulous log, I crafted the manuscript for the nursing journal. Dr. Maddern reviewed the final draft for accuracy.

Its publication resulted in several key note speeches. Heather always came along, so attendees could get a chance to see for themselves that severe deprivation does not always result in ruin.

During my second year of studies to earn a master's degree in nursing. I contacted Jeff's pulmonologist, Dr. Floyd Livingston, about an internship. For months I tagged along with him or his partner, Dr. David Geller, who described the lungs as musical instruments. "Be attuned to the sounds heard through a stethoscope; they are clues to underlying pathology," he said. He could duplicate the melody of wheezes, squeaks, stridor, whistles, rhonchi, and grating noises with exquisite and amusing accuracy.

From the two pulmonologists, I learned to suspect that my daughters had asthma.

Dr. Livingston examined Heather and Jamie at the clinic. Until then, physicians hadn't recognized their frequent bronchitis and recurrent coughing as asthma. He prescribed newly FDA-approved inhaled corticosteroid medication that assisted in healing inflamed lungs, allowing new and healthy ciliated epithelium to develop.

Asthma in severe, untreated form can result in death or a stint on a ventilator. Some of the patients transferred to the children's hospital were in critical condition. Distraught, my mentors emphasized that such distress should never have happened. Of the thousands of previously hospitalized asthmatic patients referred to them, in a year's time, only one was readmitted to the hospital. They prescribed daily preventative inhaled or oral medications and provided detailed education on asthma prevention.

After driving a ninety-minute commute, I would arrive at their office at 8:00 a.m. We first reviewed x-rays of our patients in radiology before moving on to making rounds in the neonatal intensive-care unit, general pediatrics floor, and pediatric intensive-care unit. Medical students or residents often accompanied us, and sometimes a visiting foreign doctor.

On index cards, I jotted down what Dr. Livingston asked the patients and his teachings about physical exams, testing, treatments, and medications. Some of his key inquiries: Do you cough or wheeze more than twice a week in the day? More than two times a month at night? Can you run without coughing or wheezing? How many times a year do you get bronchitis? And a standard thirty questions more, but he always concluded by teasing the kids in a happy way, "You only have one mommy, right? Take good care of her; you haven't any spares."

At lunch we went our different ways. In the afternoons, we tended to patients attending specialty clinics for cystic fibrosis, asthma, general pulmonology, or an outreach clinic to Children's Medical Services. Some of the diseases more commonly afflicting the children were sickle-cell disease, near-drowning, muscular dystrophy, asthma, and babies with coexisting congenital heart defects.

While waiting for the next patient, Dr. Livingston asked me to dictate the medical note. Dumbfounded, I remained silent, not voicing my apprehension. "You came here to learn, correct?" he prompted, followed by a quick lesson on the format and how to work the tape recorder.

On a Friday night, for a break from my graduate studies, we trailered the boat to Sebastian Inlet. Heather was then nine years old, Tony eleven, and Jamie sixteen. In a gentle mood, the river lapped against the slanting concrete boat ramp. Mangroves threw long shadows from the illuminating street lamp. Splats of whitewash-like guano dotted the dock. I sat cross-legged on weathered planks. An osprey descended out of the dark, its wings back-flapping to slow its momentum, intent on landing on a piling. Startled by my presence, it swerved toward the open river. Jim backed the trailer down the ramp until the wheels submerged.

"Did you put the plugs in?" I couldn't stop myself from asking. On land, we remove them so rainwater can drain.

"Yes," Jim answered, impatient with my insinuation of carelessness.

Though wearing a sweatshirt, Jamie complained that it was cold. On the hottest of days, once night falls and a breeze blows across the river, it feels chilly. With a hard shove, Jim sent the boat rolling into the brackish water. It bucked and bobbed before settling down into a swaying float. Jim asked Jamie to pull the slack out of the rope.

"Heather, I need more muscles!" Jamie requested. Heather sparkled at being so essential.

Jim drove the van and trailer to the parking area. He returned, jumped in the boat, and revved up the outboard motor. We all clambered in.

The propeller puttered sweetly in reverse, moving us to deeper water. Jim shifted into forward. The changing breeze had his T-shirt alternately billowing and clinging, showing off the contours of his muscular shoulders and narrow waist. Stars sparkled in the night sky. Powdery clouds drifted past a half-moon. The silhouette of the tree-lined northern shore resembled a sleeping dinosaur with a long neck, rounded spine, and elongated curving tail.

Tony shone a powerful spotlight along the shoreline. "Brrrhah," scolded a great blue heron caught in the beam, and then it took flight. Tony's displayed an intention of mischief.

"Don't blast that light ray at other boats or at your sister," Jim cautioned. "Focus it low on the water."

Heather and I scanned the illuminated surface. Chubby blue crabs drifted by, actively working all their appendages. In a clump of weeds, two tiny pairs of red specs glowed. Together Heather and I clutched the long aluminum pole and dipped the shrimping net. On deck, we dumped out two little creatures. Heather plucked up each shrimp up by its tail, and threw them in the live-well.

Toward midnight, we called it quits. Our harvest numbered only a dozen. Back at the boat ramp, there was a sight we'd never seen. About two hundred hermit crabs congregated in the shallows. They scurried about, carting their miniature homes of various-shaped shells. Some gleamed like polished pearl; others were shaggy with moss or jagged with barnacles. Smaller crabs withdrew completely into their mobile homes, but bigger ones couldn't. A fish carcass lay above the waterline. Maybe it had attracted the hermit crab festivities.

"Mom, watch the race," Tony said. He lined up four hermit crabs. Their personalities seemed to vary. One took off, covering a lot of distance. The rest remained motionless, until two middle-of-the-roaders made their move. One sought shelter; the other ambled along until he got lost in the crowd. The last one didn't budge, but nestled in, immobile.

I thanked Tony for an amusing finish for the day. Jim pulled the boat out, and we headed home.

Many children have ear, nose, and throat illnesses and disorders, so I asked Dr. Maddern to study at his clinic for my last rotation. His wife, Barbara, extended their gracious hospitality. Accepting, I stayed there for two different weeks, with a break in-between.

I knocked at their door. Looking at me through the window, their warm-hearted Labrador, Sierra, barked and wagged her tail.

"Who could it be?" I heard Bruce ask. "Oh, it's Ann." He opened the door.

"You forgot I was coming?"

Bruce, Barbara, and I gathered on the wooden stools at the center island in the kitchen. Barbara piled a mound of jalapeno-spiced boiled crawfish onto a platter. They chatted on about how they'd met and their extended families. I added my stories. Barbara told one from their early marriage when they were living in their first apartment.

"Bruce woke me in the middle of the night.

'Look,' he said, quite animated.

'What?' I asked.

'It's resting on its haunches, peering at me. A hamster. It's sitting on my chest.'

'You must be dreaming,' I mumbled, without opening my eyes.

'Missed him. I stared back at the rodent, and he scampered off, through the heating duct into the wall.'

"I gave Bruce a good razzing," Barbara paused, laughing, rubbing hilarious tears from her eyes. "Round two, the next night he roused me to receive his vindication. I saw the whiskered little animal, sitting on his nightshirt. It was the neighbor's lost pet."

Bruce Maddern hushed me on the commute to his office. "Quiet in the morning; start the day slow." I took notes as he examined patients, and then performed my own examination. I observed Dr. Maddern performing various surgeries. He quipped to the surgical team, "Be careful what you say. Ann will write it down."

To relax at the end of the day, I played with their dog, borrowed a bicycle, and swam in the pool with their children. Bruce and Barbara would cook the evening meal, or we'd go out to a local restaurant. "Ann, where are you going to work when you graduate?" Barbara asked me.

"I don't know," I answered. "But Heather still says she wants to be a surgeon like Dr. Bruce when she grows up. To do it, she'll have to figure out how to excel at standardized testing."

It bears repeating, I was agog at how life had brought me to that particular point. *Pinch my arm and wake me up.* Same as Ed had said, never in any of my imaginings had I envisioned my life and my family's to play out this way.

CHAPTER 26]
JOURNEY WITH HEART

On our friend's fiftieth birthday, his wife, Mary, threw him a surprise party. Under a cluster of palm trees, candles floated in the pool of the waterfront home. An attractive waitress paused so Jim could select some wood-skewered roasted vegetables. He'd already loaded his plate with tortilla chips and cheese dip. A conservative but voluptuous dancer entertained. The face of the man celebrating a half-century blushed at her close rendition of the traditional birthday song.

Since I was soon graduating, Mary introduced me to Dr. Mahesh Soni, a pediatrician from India. Never had I met someone from that country before. Conversation flowed easily. The hiring of a nurse-practitioner for his solo practice had become a consideration. He wrote my name down on a notepad and returned it to his pocket.

"I graduate in one month, but I'm going to Birmingham for a one-year pulmonary fellowship. They let me design my own clinical rotations with a series of pediatric subspecialty mentors. Maybe we can talk more when I return," I said.

Soon, my December graduation arrived. Jim, our children, and my parents proudly attended the ceremony. Afterward we celebrated at an Italian restaurant. Heather ordered her favorite meal, spaghetti. She'd colored me a congratulatory card.

At campus I picked up a recommendation letter from my instructor. She rummaged through a magazine to an advertised PICU nurse-practitioner position. "Sounds like you," she said. Then and there we typed a cover letter and faxed it with my resume.

Twenty-two years earlier at Florida State University, my roommate, also named Celeste, had encouraged me to switch majors from education to nursing due to a job shortage in the former. Back then, I worked weekends as a waitress at a pancake house, alongside out-of-work teachers.

Celeste happened to be vacationing in Florida and stopped to eat pizza with us on her way home. All the staff at Bizzarro's conversed in Italian. The cook hand-tossed a ball of dough into a jumbo pie. With a huge wooden paddle, he lifted the pizza's edge to check on its progress to golden perfection. We feasted on the tasty slices, each dripping mozzarella and topped with pepperoni. My friend jabbered on about her life.

Back home, making coffee in the kitchen, Jim pushed the playback button on the answering machine. The message rendered us speechless: "Hello Ann. This is Dr. Kris Bysani. I am an intensivist and the director of the pediatric intensive-care unit at the Children's Hospital of Illinois. I'd like to discuss the possibility of flying you here for an interview. We are a quiet people, mostly farmers. Many parents prefer our locale to Chicago or St. Louis. If you would kindly call me at your earliest convenience."

I'd forgotten about faxing that application with my professor. Timing was perfect, as Birmingham had just notified me that they'd lost their funding and cancelled my fellowship. A recruiter booked my flight to Peoria and reserved a room at the city's best hotel. For three days, I had hourly interviews with all the key people, and dinners in the evenings. I'd mailed them my airway-suction research paper ahead of time. When the whirlwind meetings were done, they offered me a position, and I accepted.

Venturing to Illinois on my own; Jim tucked the last medical book into the trunk of my car. Arriving safely, I checked into the same hotel that I'd stayed in for the interviews. The PICU at the Children's Hospital of Illinois in Peoria treated every kind of critical illness afflicting children and specialized in correcting congenital heart defects. Every year, two hundred fifty babies and children underwent heart surgery at their expert facility.

Each cardiac patient seemed a miracle. Earlier in my career, when techniques for surgical correction had not yet been developed, the outcome was always tragic. Babies with cyanotic congenital heart defects became bluer and bluer until they died.

On my first day of work, I hoped a poker face disguised my shock. A PICU nurse lifted a cloth lying on a young baby's chest. I stared at his splayed-open sternum and beating heart, only covered by a thin, transparent surgical dressing. I felt a visceral fear, as I never knew of such things. What if something fell off my person and onto the fragile beating organ? What if I tripped?

The nurse gently palpated the baby's fingers and toes to check for warmth and looked for pink color. Both being normal indicated an appropriate mix of medications and assisted ventilation had been prescribed to promote good blood circulation. In a day or two, when tissue swelling decreased, the surgeon would cinch the sternal wires taut to draw the breastbone closed, then seal the skin with a series of stitches. The baby's heart would again be protected by the rib cage.

Babies undergoing complex heart surgery begin the recovery period with a tube in their mouth to their airway. An electronic ventilator gives them breaths. Their bodies are invaded multi-fold by numerous intravenous lines dripping medications, chest tubes, surgical drains, temporary pacemaker wires, and numerous laboratory draws.

I endeavored to learn the art, thought process, and factual calculation of drugs, drips, ventilator and pacemaker settings, nutrition, labs, and radiology. Studies consumed all my waking moments. Mornings began with 6:30 a.m. multispecialty rounds where we stopped at each patient's bedside to review and modify care. The base team was comprised of an intensivist, pediatric cardiac surgeon, cardiologist, nutritionist, charge nurse, and me. Some days the group included a general surgeon, neurologist, orthopedist, urologist, and/or nephrologist. They all taught me. I felt like the luckiest person alive.

At the same time, I was so very homesick. Sometimes I called my father, sobbing like when I was a young girl. Dad encouraged perseverance. Jim spoiled me with letters and creative gifts. To alleviate my loneliness, Jim booked flights for Tony and Heather to join me for the remainder of the year. So Jim wouldn't get stricken with aloneness, and as Jamie was a senior in high school, she would remain in Florida with Jim.

In preparation, I rented a house near a middle school. The spaciousness and novelty of a basement frightened me, maybe Bigfoot slept there. I kept that door bolted. A little stream trickled across the back of the steeply sloped lot. Without the benefit of any caretaking, tomatoes sprouted and prospered in its clay soil. In my bedroom, I slept on an air mattress and sleeping bag.

By the time Tony and Heather joined me, Illinois was cold. We rarely felt warm and relished having several gas fireplaces. At bedtime we cranked up the one in the living room, spread out our sleeping bags, and slept close to it.

On a meager budget, we lived without furniture or television. We sat on the floor or on bench seats that were part of the built-in wall shelving. A house-wide intercom music system played the tunes of our favorite radio stations.

Intensivist Drs. Al Torres and Kris Bysani shared their vast knowledge of pulmonary issues. Together we established an outpatient clinic for tracheotomy and ventilator-dependent pediatric patients and revamped the pediatric advanced life support (PALS) course.

Whether he would be on duty or have the day off, Dr. Torres reviewed each upcoming cardiac surgical case—its standard treatment and potential complications. He emphasized to use caution and not to blindly accept other subspecialty recommendations due to their more narrowed focus on one body system. Well-intentioned guidance might harm the patient. For example, discontinuing ventilator assistance too soon can result in pulmonary hemorrhage.

Surprisingly, Dr. Torres relished intense questioning of his approach to treatment. "I like losing an argument," he said. "It means I learn something new."

Weekends were for exploring Chicago or enjoying one of the many small farm-town festivals. On Friday nights, we headed to the movies. Indulgent, we ordered a refillable tub of buttered popcorn and ate two. Stunt-biking at the dirt race-course was a frequent leisure activity. Tony and Heather jumped and hit berms and rode whoopty-doos (popping wheelies off small bumps on the track). Wipeouts didn't squash their enthusiasm. For a sweet treat, we'd enjoy a dish of "Moo-newer" ice cream at the local parlor. Amusing name.

My father booked a flight to visit. In preparation we made garage-sale purchases of a couch for him to sleep on and a ping-pong table. At Thanksgiving, Jim and my mother came. For the festivities, we acquired a dining table and matching chairs. Since Bigfoot never materialized, the basement became our hang-out with fast games of ping-pong, snacks in its refrigerator, and supplies for crafts.

As a hobby, Heather wove hemp bracelets with knots and beads. She created a special one for a teenager who'd undergone a kidney transplant and was suffering severe complications. Heather wrote a caring note, then visited in person to give her the bracelet and a salmon-pink queen conch shell. The two new friends took turns holding it to their ears and listening for the ocean.

That brave teenager had dreams of visiting the Atlantic seashore when she got well. Tragically, she died. At the funeral, Heather and I were standing with the mother by the open casket when the mother gently lifted her deceased daughter's wrist and removed the hemp bracelet. "Suzy would never take it off," she said, then the mother asked that Heather tie the bracelet to the mother's own wrist. We offered our condolences.

Lest I be remiss, I should mention that doctors cry. The best of them, the most expert of them, I have seen them cry. As the years go by, it happens less often, as it is difficult to do this kind of work and have the tears flow.

Heather had a new idea for what she wanted to be when she grew up, after getting to know the nurses that cared for Suzy, she thought she might want to become a nurse.

When the year in Peoria was up, Tony, Heather, and I moved back home. I thought about searching for employment at another big-city hospital, but my good friend disagreed.

"You know enough," Karen said. "Call Dr. Soni. Physicians from India are smart. I've met him. He's a good man." I dialed his secretary. He interviewed me the same morning. Afterward we lunched with the staff. One more meeting, and I joined his pediatrics practice as a nurse practitioner. The next day, he left for a three-week vacation in India. "No patients while I am gone. Read the charts; review the thicker ones. It is a good way to learn," he said.

When he returned, I shadowed him for one month and took notes. Mahesh Soni spoke quietly and briefly in the accent of his country. Sometimes patients had difficulty understanding him. He is short for an American, but tall for his ethnicity and broad-shouldered.

Each work day began at the hospital as a physician/nurse-practitioner team writing our progress notes and examining newborn babies and hospitalized children. Our set schedule consisted of alternating between our two offices, each working on our own. We switched in the middle of the day, stopping by home for lunch. "Consult with me over the telephone if you're unsure of a diagnosis or treatment," he said. One afternoon a week, we continued to work together in the same office so he could teach me directly.

Dr. Soni exuded quiet excellence. Before anyone spoke, before performing any hands-on physical examination, he usually knew the diagnosis by observing the patients—their behavior, posture, how they breathed, moved, and color of their skin. He was living proof of the adage; "Ask questions to confirm observations; examine to verify illness history given by the patient; and order tests only if needed to pinpoint a different diagnosis and treatment."

I could search the medical literature for days, and never find the information that I sought. When I gave up and questioned Dr. Soni, he would summarize the answer in a few key words. In the office he was businesslike, working quickly and efficiently. On occasion, he'd grace us with sudden humor and melodious laughter. He told me about one of his first experiences in this country, walking in downtown New York City.

"'Hey, Gandhi!' a stranger called out to me," Soni said. "Naïve, I thought the man had questions about Gandhi and India's independence movement, but my friend corrected me. The guy was robbing me of my wallet and watch. I handed them over."

"Welcome to America," was his friend's wry comment.

Every other Saturday morning, to give most of our staff off, I worked with one medical assistant who had to be secretary and nurse. Heather would come with me to clinic. Twelve years old, she'd help answer phones, catch up the filing, and hand out stickers to the patients.

Procrastination ended. Heather and I stopped by the hospital lab for her to have a sweat test to quantify its salt content. I'd mentioned a nagging concern to Dr. Soni. "Heather has symptoms of cystic fibrosis, but I don't want to know. I prefer to be blissfully ignorant."

"If you test her, and the result is negative, you will gain peace of mind," he wisely advised.

The technician strapped a device on Heather's forearm and left it for thirty minutes to collect her perspiration. The lab determined the salt percentage. It was normal, no cystic fibrosis.

Life went smoothly for a couple of years, and then it didn't. Devastating news came our way.

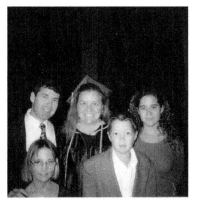

Ann's graduation from University of Central Florida's Nurse Practioner, MSN, master of science in nursing program.

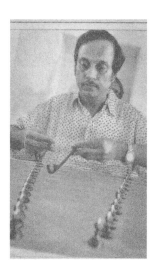

Dr. Mahesh Soni, pediatrician,
Playing the santoor

CHAPTER 27]
DEVASTATING NEWS

The news of 2001 prodded us to find faith, hope, and laughter in adversity. Heather, whom Jim had so carefully tended during her fragile years, began quietly watching over her dad. Jim had just turned forty-eight years old. Vibrant Heather was fourteen, boisterous Tony was sixteen, and Jamie was twenty-one and a student studying marine biology at Florida Tech, where still Jim worked in the computer department overseeing the business aspects of the school.

Prior to the news that swallowed us whole, a lesser, recurring difficulty reared its head. Heather had once again failed the annual reading FCAT (Florida Comprehensive Assessment Test). Without eventually passing the three-hour exam, Florida rules disallowed her graduation from high school. No high-school diploma, just a certificate of attendance.

Mandatory remedial classes and their too simple material bored her silly. She knew reading; she just had difficulty with the structure of that test. Failing the FCAT prohibited her from taking the regular reading curriculum. Her knowledge began slipping behind that of her peers. Year after year, Heather had always applied herself to her schoolwork and achieved final grades of A or B on her report card. The repeated FCAT failure left her in a quandary.

She had no idea what she might pursue as a career, or could, if a single test could close the door to a college education.

In September, the terrible news began this way. Feeling very ill, Jim thought a stomach virus gripped him. Painful spasms prompted teasing that perhaps he was giving birth. His doctor ordered some blood tests. Dr. Soni's wife worked in the hospital lab. "Mahesh, what is wrong with Ann's Jim?" Rita Soni asked. She calculated that Jim's white blood cell count exceeded 50,000. Tests determined he suffered from chronic lymphocytic leukemia and small cell lymphoma. Lymph nodes as large as fruit in his abdomen impeded blood flowing in his major arteries.

Slow and insidious cancers, unknown to us, they had subtly afflicted him for awhile before orchestrating catastrophe. In hindsight, we could recognize how the disease had been affecting him, fatigue, less enthusiasm, not wanting to go to the beach. Photographs where his skin tones were too white.

The day of diagnosis, too numb to think, out of necessity, I instantly became stronger than steel and as carefree as bubbles floating on the wind. Even among enormous tribulations, ever-present joys persist and thread through the troubles like trickles of gold hidden in a mountain. Simple things like silliness, random smiles, walking the dog, crock-pot soup, prayer, yoga, sunsets, and the ocean gained even greater importance.

Amidst the sorrows, family life chugged Jim and I forward with the responsibility of parenting of two teenagers and a university student, though most of that fell on my shoulders. My work load at the pediatrics practice accelerated as the number of patients we cared for steadily increased. I kept up my busy schedule of five or six days a week, plus taking calls by phone every other night. Lack of time thwarted any chance of sinking into self-pity. Grudgingly, I accepted the saying, "and why not my family?"

In the wee hours, Jim's non-stop hacking woke me. "It's difficult to breathe. A glob of mucous is obstructing my throat," he said. His voice sounded peculiar and terrified. Its pitch changed to resemble the voice of Donald Duck.

"Please don't. That isn't mucous. It is your epiglottis, a flap of tissue that moves to cover the windpipe when swallowing," I said. "If it continues to swell, it'll get too large and obstruct your airway."

Jim couldn't abide my suggestion and continued trying to cough up his own throat. Straining for oxygen, he shifted his posture into the ominous triangle-pose, the only position that kept his airway open. He sat leaning forward with his hands on his knees, neck stretched out, nose strained out.

Scribbling a white lie to the children that we left early to take the car to the repair shop, I drove Jim to the emergency room, purposefully opting against an ambulance. If a technician erred in his judgement and ignored my cautions, he might look into Jim's mouth. Such a manipulation would likely cause a quick progression to a complete and fatal airway obstruction.

On our arrival, an emergency room doctor assessed Jim. "Does he always sound like Donald Duck?"

"Of course not," I replied. Epiglottitis has become infrequent with today's vaccines. Most medical personnel have never seen a case.

An otolaryngologist examined Jim and made preparations for creating a tracheotomy in Jim's neck if the airway obstruction worsened. Next to arrive were his cancer and family practice doctors. Radiology, blood samples, meds, intravenous fluids; yeah, he remained stable. A nurse moved him into a wheelchair and transferred him to the intensive care unit. I followed along. She stuck cardiorespiratory monitors to his chest. Screens displayed information about his vital processes. Hmm, we had done this before. Once he seemed settled, I drove to the office.

Amazing, I arrived on-time for the first patient's appointment at 9:00 a.m. No one could substitute and tend to the numerous children that I assisted, nor generate my portion of the income that went toward paying our office overhead and payroll, which included my paycheck. Essential if Jim couldn't work or passed on. Each morning before work and afterward every evening, I went to Jim. For my health, I always slept at home.

Heather insisted on sitting at her dad's side during the day, and ushered him strength. Her hand sponged Jim's forehead with a cool wash cloth. With my guidance, her eyes and ears became extensions of mine. Mustering politeness and assertiveness, she requested copies of his labs and radiology reports. Over the phone, she read me the names of medicines dissolved in the bags of fluid that dripped into his vein. She scanned his monitors. How uncanny and beautiful that Heather would traverse the difficult road with Jim, her siblings, and me.

Side-effects of chemotherapy infusions tempered Christmas and New Year's Day celebrations. Jim forged ahead in the best, festive mood that he could muster, despite nausea, difficult breathing, fatigue, and belly pain. He forced himself to eat to survive. He managed a few feeble smiles. He grew grumpy. The kids and I faked toughness on that. We cared for him without cowering to his every whim, stifling any temptation to smother with too much indulgence. The approach was a gift from us—to always propagate his dignity.

After a year, he achieved a small remission. When the reprieve ended, we kept the struggle mostly private. Jim didn't like the daily strangeness that came with people knowing of his cancer. Immediate family members and select co-workers helped him weather the on-going storms.

It was fortunate that Jim had changed out of the grocery business. Otherwise he couldn't have contributed financially to the family, as the job of a store manager is too physically strenuous. Thank goodness for the profession of computer analyst and the dignity it provided.

Jim's boss was flexible. She let him not work, or work from office or home: short days, weekend days. He had years of accumulated sick leave. His paycheck was steady. In weeks of more energy, he could work some extra hours, to accumulate for when he took off. Though fatigue, coughing, discomfort, nausea, and difficulty breathing often taxed him, his mind remained sharp. The months he had random pain or was too weak to drive, a coworker or one of the children would drive him.

Jim wasn't the only one doing poorly. Meagan, our oldest Scotty dog, no longer moved from the rug to greet us. Instead of a vigorous wag, her tail barely swished the floor. Tony petted her head. "Mom, her fur is turning gray. Nessie will be so lonely. For my birthday, can we get a puppy?"

"Maybe another Scottish terrier from a litter of one of her pups?" I suggested.

"How about a bigger breed, like a pit bull?" Tony asked.

"Perhaps something less controversial, such as a Labrador or boxer?" Jim replied.

On our way to the grocery store, we spied a yard sign advertising boxer pups. All were claimed except a small, plump male. Mamma dog blessed me with kisses and wagged not just her tail, but her whole body. Jim phoned Jamie and asked her to help us surprise Tony and Heather. "Invite them for ice cream, but drive here instead."

When our three children arrived, the breeder opened the door to his slightly stinky back-porch and several litters of puppies. Their eldest son baulked at treading among the poop to retrieve the pup. No need, the fat, little male boxer waddled in and padded over to Tony. They became instantly smitten. The pup was a toffee color, with a splash of white on his chest and the tips of his paws. Tony named him Tank.

Two weeks later, we brought him home. Confining Tank in a dog crate or the hall bathroom failed. Claustrophobic, he would thrash about and soil his bedding. Letting him freely roam the house seemed a safer alternative. When tired, he would curl up amidst the stuffed animals on Heather's lowest bookcase shelf and take a nap.

Half a year later, Tank weighed fifty pounds. In the wee hours of one morning, Tank whined at each of our beds until we wakened. He bade us to follow along to old dog Meagan, who twitched with a seizure. Jim, Jamie, Tony, Heather, and I kept vigil on the floor by her pillow bed. Spunky Nessie seemed oblivious and begged for attention by dropping off an array of dog toys. Sweet old dog Meagan passed on.

Tony dug a deep hole under the cedar trees and layered it with soft branches. Jamie and Heather dropped in orange hibiscus flowers. Before lowering Meagan in a basket, we formed a circle, clasped hands, and recited a few prayers. Tank and Nessie sat at our feet. A sudden thought had us halt the ceremony.

"Witnessing the burial might give Tank and Nessie nightmares. They'll not understand," Tony said. Into the house with the dogs, then we lowered Meagan and each took turns shoveling in sand to cover the lifeless pet.

After Meagan's passing, the boxer and younger Scotty wouldn't sleep solo. They nestled close, even when growing Tank topped a muscular one-hundred pounds. Always joyous in his greetings, just the way his mamma had, Tank licked at the air and waggled his whole body. For the fun of it, during one of the kids' games, he leapt over the volleyball net without snagging any of his paws. He would also hurdle our six-foot wooden fence, just because he could, and drop into the neighbor's yard.

Heather destined me to plunge ever deeper into not only studying about otolaryngology for the benefit of my patients, but also having to live it. Lounging on the couch, Heather said, "My left ear keeps oozing. It's clear and gooey like jellyfish guts. Smell it," she said, laughing at her crassness and underlying apprehension. She waved a dab of it stuck on the tip of her little finger near to my nose.

"Yuck." I said, and made an icky face. "Perhaps it is a swimmer's-ear infection."

When it persisted despite treatment, Dr. Soni examined Heather's ear with an otoscope. Exudate made it difficult to visualize the eardrum. He suspected a cholesteotoma (an erosive mass that infects the middle ear and mastoid bone). Unchecked, it eats at the affected ear structures and muffles hearing until the sense is completely lost. Without surgical treatment, if both ears become diseased, complete deafness is the end result. Surrounded by silence, cut off from spoken words, a person eventually loses all ability to talk.

With the images of the CAT scan of her left ear and temporal bone, we headed to Jacksonville. Dr. Maddern concurred with Dr. Soni's diagnosis. The thought of Heather under-going anesthesia, intubation, and surgery frightened Jim and me. Would her trachea become damaged and scar? I tried not to worry about the possibility of her again needing a tracheotomy.

Raising Heather always propelled Jim and me toward a more mystical and less intellectual approach to life. Indian culture and its spirituality veered us toward newer perceptions. With Heather's upcoming operation, an invitation to a three-day program on prayer at the Hindu temple rang fortuitous. Mahesh and Rita Soni drove me the first evening. Mom came along for the second; Jim accompanied me on the third.

An old frame house near the river served as the temple. As their custom, we removed our shoes and left them outside on their porch. Greetings and exchanging names followed, but the unfamiliar Hindi syllables made them difficult to retain. A slow-moving, shiny black beetle crawled across a table. An elderly man gently slid notepaper underneath and cupped his hand around, to release it outside.

His wife, with her long hair woven into an intricate braid, expressed an interest in how we came to attend. She offered some insights, explaining that Hindus believe in only one God as a formless energy. "*Bhagvan* is the Hindi word for God," she said. Yet many devotees can better contemplate divine energy when God is presented in varying forms. Some can comprehend a fat and happy god, or a scary one hoisting a big sword, or a musical and married god. These additional gods seem akin to the saints, to whom Christians offer prayers.

Ladies in traditional saris sat cross-legged upon the floor on cushioned, white sheets on the right side of the room. The men sat in a similar fashion on the left. The celebration progressed with rituals of candles, incense, traditional Indian music, and Hindu prayers. Translations seemed familiar and similar to the common Christian prayers.

"Praise God, calling him what you want: Jesus, Yahweh, Krishna, Buddha, Allah. The name is not important," Swami Shantanandnand said in opening. He elaborated on the main theme of worshiping God, with or without form. The devoted man had travelled from south India and had studied under world-renowned Swami Chinmayananda.

A few words were spoken in Sanskrit, though most teaching was in English. Swami spoke of issues common to all people. I remember those that resonated strongly:

Marriage, Swami spoke on loving one's spouse and Marriage: For a few weeks, a man tries to be a partner's dream image, before becoming his true self. Joy materializes in the loving of the real person, not the dream.

Faith, Swami spoke on the testing and questioning of Faith: Faith in God may be easy while enjoying young love, until a tragedy—perhaps the beautiful wife dies. The grieving husband may falter in his faith and rant, "Why her, God? Why not an old woman? Why not a wicked one?"

Prayer, Swami spoke on true Prayer versus just going through the motions: A villager prayed to Durga three hours a day for many months, but was not fully sincere. One day, he lit incense to entice the god to show herself. When the smoke drifted toward Ganesh, he accused the elephant god of thievery.

"Why do you steal Durga's incense?" As the villager hurled his rants at Ganesh, the elephant god materialized as a form that could be seen. The villager fussed even louder. "All these years I pray to Durga, and never does she manifest. But never have I prayed to you; why did you come to me?"

"Because in your sincere reprimanding of me, you demonstrated a true belief in my existence," Ganesh explained.

Infinite God, Swami spoke on the universal presence of The Infinite God: A true believer rested his feet on a statue of the deity, Hanuman.

"That is disrespectful," his friend commanded.

"Where can I place my feet that there is not God?" the believer asked. Nevertheless, the man moved his feet as bidden. Every new place that he set his toes upon the ground, there again, Hanuman sprang up beneath them. His friend stared in amazement and contemplated the significance of his friend's words. God is everywhere.

At the completion of the teaching, all partook in small plates of blessed food and enjoyed other refreshments. Jim browsed an educational display and purchased a few booklets. A middle-aged man began sweeping the floor. We bid our farewells.

Refreshed with newer tools and an expanding vision of faith, we scheduled Heather's surgery in hopes of preserving her hearing. Cholesteotoma, even when treated, has a high rate of recurrence.

A chest x-ray taken prior to surgery revealed a miracle had transpired. Heather's lungs looked perfect. They'd renewed themselves with no traces of the multitude of previous abnormalities.

Essential for medical miracles to happen is that the critical "C" of choice exists—freedom to choose or dismiss a physician, seek an additional opinion, or to be examined by a specialist. Pediatric subspecialists had restored Heather's health, abated lingering illness, and avoided unnecessary, repetitive, and costly interventions; and we hoped, would preserve her hearing.

Pediatric pulmonology. Voilà! an appointment with Dr. Livingston, who prescribed one preventative medication, and Heather's lungs transcended all injuries. She rarely had asthma symptoms, no pulmonary hospitalizations, and no missed school days. When asked whether she could run or participate in sports? The answer had become a resounding yes to sprinting, and yes to any athletics.

Pediatric otolaryngology. Airway reconstructive surgery by Dr. Maddern had generated the miracles of producing speech and a splashing capacity to swim. Every day we rejoiced at her spoken words. How glorious that she could dive under an ocean wave and glide with the eagle rays at Molasses Reef.

Pediatrics. Care by an excellent pediatrician, protector of all facets of children's health. Dr. Soni's recognition of Heather's very diseased left ear prevented serious complicating infection, such as often-killer meningitis. He'd judiciously referred further care to Dr.

Maddern, who would work hard to preserve her hearing—a sense especially dear to otolaryngologists.

Sometimes the system fails sick children. Maybe an essential second or third medical opinion never materializes, perhaps as a consequence of insurance restrictions or "gatekeeping," financial issues, simple ignorance, or referring to a good-politics doctor instead of the best for the patient. Other failures are a result of doctors who provide superficial care, because the patients have little option to go elsewhere.

Due to low reimbursement, most physicians refused treatment of Medicaid patients, as seeing one often costs the doctor money, instead of generating income. Some salaried doctors, who work at clinics that accept Medicaid patients, get lazy and turn them away. They will receive the same amount of money in their paycheck whether they treat hundreds of patients or almost none at all.

Another potential source of calamity is misdiagnosis. The featured speaker at the American Society of Pediatric Otolaryngology's dinner gala had grown up in a mental institution. Comedy was the medium the young woman utilized to get her message across. At a young age, she'd been erroneously labeled as severely retarded. Her real trouble was profound deafness. Later as an adult, she was injured in a car accident and told that she would never again walk.

"I grew tired of physician predictions confining me," she said. "I decided to strive for what the doctors had dubbed impossible: an education, spoken language, and ambulation. Though I couldn't hear, I learned to communicate through lip-reading and responding with my own voice. With guidance, my legs grew strong and took tentative steps. I banished the wheelchair." That evening, we witnessed her beautiful success.

Dr. Maddern confirmed that the sad scenario still occurred. Recently he'd diagnosed an older child with previously unrecognized profound deafness. "Universal screening of all newborns for an ability to hear should reduce such tragic oversights in the future," he said.

CHAPTER 28]
PRESERVING HEARING

The blending scents of surgical scrub, antibiotics, and not-quite-well perspiration seemed forever etched into my nostrils and memory. Carved there and suppressed, painful scents and images, no longer pressed there solely through caring for Heather, but also my Jim. Dreams for her seemed always to come true. My dreams for married life with Jim shattered. As in the analogy, we'd landed in another country, and it too had its richness.

The kids and I weathered the ups and downs of Jim's illness and adjusted to his diminished vigor. When he took chemo infusions, Heather drove him and remained at his side. I couldn't, as I was working. The cancer and newer chemotherapy damaged his lungs. Often his mother, who lived near Florida Tech, would pick him up at work and take him to her home for lunch and a nap, then drive him back to work.

More and more he dialed in to the work network from home. Some weeks he lingered all day on the couch on our sunny back porch, content just to breathe. We looked for time, not a miracle. He'd take a little treatment to carry him to the next family vacation or graduation.

Most times, he chose the treatment that had been around the longest, chlorambucil pills by mouth, to keep the proliferation of white cells in his blood at bay. The number of them would grow so large as to turn his blood to sludge and his skin to white. Chlorambucil beat back the cancer and was easiest on his body. Never a cure, but some reprieve. Maybe he'd survive to see one or our children marry and hold our first grandchild.

No drug regimen provided a cure. Many proved more damaging than the cancer. His oncologist had difficulty with the concept of not administering more anti-cancer drugs. He wished to be doing something concrete. But the doctor did not walk with all Jim's suffering. I reminded the oncologist of "Do No Harm" and the age-old question that just because something can be done, should it be done? How is that determined?

When reaching for the improbable, the radiation doctor turned us down, saying it would not benefit Jim. Sometimes I wondered if we'd done right by Jim. Perhaps he should never have taken any chemo at all. We kept doing the best we could with the imperfect information and systems available. I turned to prayer. There is always the ripple effect. Jim the man and his fight to survive impacted the university and the children and me in many profound and on-going ways.

Another worry.

Heather's need for ear surgery. The potential for new airway scarring and tracheotomy terrified Jim and me. To avoid airway damage, the anesthesiologist would insert a smaller-sized intubation tube than usual. Behind Heather's ear drum, growths encased the three little bones and snuffed the hearing in her left ear. Cholesteotomas are dangerous. They keep spreading and can penetrate into the brain, often creating fatal infection.

"There aren't many more parts of your ears and throat to operate on," Dr. Maddern said to Heather. Both seemed bemused at the comment. He was talking to us in the before-surgery holding area. Older now, I would no longer hold her in my arms as she wafted off to sleep.

A nurse wheeled her away to surgery. I set to biding the wait in the family room. Jim had stayed at home. I did not attempt my fake reading, instead I pretend-dozed in a twilight state. Hours passed. I stopped looking at the clock. The operation was taking much longer than anticipated. No one had alerted me as to why. It would turn out however it turned out. I continued to fake sleep.

"Heather is fine," Dr. Maddern said when he finally emerged. "Most cholesteotomas are solid and simpler to remove. But instead, in Heather's middle ear, a spiderweb-like growth threaded around her hearing bones and penetrated further into the mastoid in her skull." For hours, he had tediously picked out the stringy webs. In addition, he enlarged and sculpted her left ear canal, which was congenitally extra bony and too small.

To avert infection, Dr. Maddern prescribed intravenous antibiotics twice a day for three weeks. He arranged for me to administer them to Heather at home, instead of taking her to an infusion center. "Buy some spray-in, comb-out shampoo. No water-washing her hair for one month," Maddern instructed.

A nurse transported her from the recovery room, and we got her settled into the hospital room. Layers of gauze wound around her head. It held in place a soft cup positioned to cover her ear and protect it from accidental bumps. Later that evening, Heather decided to tackle walking to the bathroom without waking me.

"Mom. Help! My legs are like jello," she croaked. I opened my eyes and saw her, dressed in a faded blue hospital gown that hung slightly parted, exposing her derriere. Her back swayed and buckled further. I lurched off the cot and reached her in time to grip her wobbly torso. She mustered some last tidbits of energy.

"No more attempting to get around on your own," I scolded, and proceeded to escort her onward to the toilet. Leaning on me for support, her skin sweated that old, familiar sick smell. Heather's legs trembled as she stood, washing her hands at the sink. Looking up from her shaky fingers and swaying balance, she inspected her reflection in the mirror. "Yikes! You should have warned me. My hair is sticking out every which way, and there's blood!" Heather recoiled at the sight of herself.

Dried blood splatters speckled her nose and cheeks. Enlarging, red stains soaked through the wraps of gauze. A few drops trickled down her ear lobe and along the lean creases of her neck.

"Don't fret. You are okay," I said.

She oh-so-slowly wet the corner of a washcloth and dabbed clean the crusty splotches. Shuffling her way back to bed, my left arm kept hold around her waist. With my right, I grasped and pulled along the rolling intravenous-fluid pole, careful not to snag the IV tubing in the wheels. All proceeded uneventfully.

Back home again, I peeled off the soiled bandages one layer at a time until I could cleanse the skin underneath. I squirted antibiotic drops onto packing tucked into the ear canal to keep it open during healing. Concerned that wayward strands of hair might contaminate her surgical wounds with infection, I divided her thick tresses into a multitude of tiny sections and wove them into individual braids. Heather selected brilliantly colored elastic bands to secure the ends. Around her head I wound fresh gauze, securing the soft protective cup in place over her tender left ear.

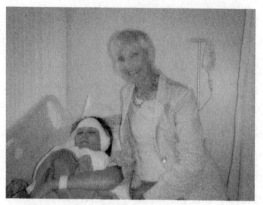

Heather and her Grandy Kathi

Annoyed is a polite understatement of how I felt about the messages left on the answering machine. The high school attendance clerk was threatening to fail Heather for nonattendance. The school board had enacted a new, no-exception policy. Any student missing more than fifteen days failed. Medical reasons or family emergencies were penalized as harshly as skipping school for a lazy day at the beach.

The clerk insisted that she would fail Heather irrespective of a medical excuse and her successful completion of all make-up work and exams. Too much, I lost my composure and loudly quoted Heather's legal right to an education. Fortunately, the school board abolished the experiment after one year and reinstated the distinction between excused and unexcused absences, but it hadn't happened yet.

Feeling strong enough to return half-days, Heather checked in at the high school's front office and handed them Dr. Maddern's written medical excuse confirming surgery. The office staff gawked at Heather's gauze-wrapped head and the plastic protective device covering her left ear. They stared at the adjacent scalp shaven of hair and the reddened and healing stitch-scarred incision lines. They chose to overlook the unfair policy and let Heather proceed to class.

Return to ROTC (Reserve Officers Training Corps) class and its drills was postponed until the completion of the three weeks of intravenous antibiotics. It seemed better to wait until I removed the venous access catheter lodged into a large arm vein. The teacher glared at her braids and growled. "Your hair must be pulled into a bun. Since it is not, I am dropping your class grade from a B to a C."

"I have a doctor's note," she said.

"A physician recommended wearing your hair in braids?" he asked.

"Please review the note," Heather urged. The letter confirmed undergoing ear and mastoid skull surgery. It explained how a bun loosens, especially when sleeping. Braids kept hair strands out of her healing incisions until mended enough to resume shampooing with water in the shower.

The instructor's mood lightened as he read. "Okay," he concluded. "Just swap out the colored elastics to brown ones that will disappear into your brunette hair."

Belting out the next admonishment came from a volunteer at the after-church youth group. When Heather didn't respond to her question, the volunteer's voice rose into a shriek. "What's the matter with you? Are you deaf? Have you cotton in your ears?"

"As a matter of fact, that is correct on both counts. I am deaf in my left ear, and there is cotton in it from recent surgery, but I have a good-hearing right ear. If you talk on my right side, I'll hear your words."

The most amusing comment came from a stranger. Once Heather was fully healed, she and Robyn and one other friend went to the beach. Walking down the beach in their bikinis, they paused to admire an elaborate sandcastle. In the sunshine, Heather's surgical scars glistened more prominently than her smooth, tanned skin.

A thick linear scar streaked downward from her upper chest and passed through her bellybutton. The old feeding-tube site bubbled up as a rounded scar. A zigzag scar marked her right chest where Maddern had harvested the rib cartilage graft. Near to it, a bean-sized scar dimpled the site where she once sported a chest tube. Puckering the mid-front of her neck was the scar from the old lifesaving tracheotomy tube.

A skinny middle-aged Jamaican man with long dreadlocks slowed to a stop as he was passing by. He apprised Heather and posed a sincere question. "Were you shot and stabbed?"

"Yes," Heather replied, deadpan, and said nothing more.

Tired from many years of questioning, she didn't bother to correct his impression.

The three girls scampered down the beach and skipped through the incoming surf. The water grew deeper, and they dove under a breaking wave, swimming through its roughness to the calm beneath. The girls surfaced, giggling non-stop.

"Let's fabricate a more exotic story for the next inquisitive stranger," Robyn suggested. The three friends carried on with great amusement as they concocted a gamut of wild and implausible explanatory scenarios. Ran into a cactus, spilled into rapids, surprised a wolf, met an alien, too many paint balls.

Complaints directed at Heather resumed when she began working at McDonald's.

Heather's spoken words sounded muffled because she barely moved her lips. She stopped way short of the precise tongue-and-lip movements needed for clear enunciation. The habit seemed a carry-over from the years she couldn't use her mouth to eat or speak. Friends and family understood her speech, so she didn't care.

"I got the job. Orientation is on Friday!" Heather effused, excited at the prospect of earning some money. For the first month, almost no customers remarked, then five complained about her voice in one day. Arriving home, she removed her greasy sneakers and left them in the garage to prevent having fast-food odors permeate her closet. She'd worked the counter that day, instead of running the grill.

"After paying for his meal, some old guy refused to take his food order. 'You're contagious,' he taunted, going on and on, making a big scene. I understand his concern, but he didn't have to be mean. I told him that my voice was normal for me and further elaborated, blah, blah, blah. 'Are you sure?' he questioned. He did eventually let me serve him his Big Mac.

"Usually a simple 'no, I am not ill' suffices. I like working the grill better than the counter. Flipping burgers and dipping hundreds of pounds of french fries into oil is a welcome respite from rude, tiresome remarks."

Customer grumbling increased exponentially when she began handling the drive-through microphone. "Use it as an opportunity to polish your speech," Jim offered in support. And she did. Heather put into action all the lessons practiced in her early years of speech therapy. Complaints dwindled to a tolerable number.

Heather was a high school senior, in her last semester. Late afternoon, she burst through the front door full of ecstatic energy. "I get to graduate! I passed the bleeping FCAT reading test by two points, two points," she chanted, pulsing the air with two outstretched fingers, the gesture similar to the well-known sign for peace. "Two lousy points, minuscule and giant, determine my whole future." She'd failed all FCAT reading tests of the previous seven years. Success just shy of the final bell, Heather felt thrilled for earning the green light to strive for greater things and infuriated that one section of a single exam could invalidate thirteen years of school attendance and successful studies.

Clad in a traditional white graduation gown, underneath Heather wore a stylish fitted dress trimmed in pink. Bright, blue skies on a hot summer day, the class of 2006 sat on fold-out chairs on the turf of Melbourne High School's football stadium. The master of ceremonies broadcast Heather's name over the loud speaker. Heather strode toward the podium and stepped across a plain wooden bridge to receive her diploma. With great pride, Jim and I, Jamie, Tony, and her grandparents stood up and cheered. The band played a celebratory song. Along with her classmates, Heather tossed her tassled cap high in the air. The symbols of achievement came drifting back down like confetti.

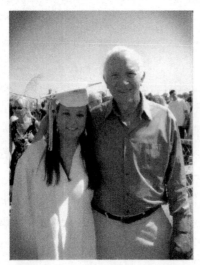

Heather and her Granddad Fritz
Melbourne High School Graduation

Afterward at a graduation party at our home, my mom served slices of carrot cake to the guests. Heather's friends decorated her old beater car with streamers and cans. On the windshield they scrawled happy words of encouragement, lettered in toothpaste.

Mahesh and Rita Soni stopped by with a gift. Heather told them about a course she was studying to become certified to perform hearing tests. Completion of the innovative CPOP (certified personnel for otolaryngology practice) program would let her perform them under the supervision of an ear, nose, and throat surgeon. "I'll attend college full-time and work part-time for my Uncle Mike," Heather said.

"If you work for a relative, he may yell at you," Mahesh said.

"Heather is a clever girl. She will know how to handle him," Rita said.

"But no need, my Uncle Mike is a sweetheart," Heather spoke the truth.

That fall, Heather enrolled at the local community college. Jim and I insisted that she pay the tuition, as such an arrangement provided her greater incentive to succeed. Her first courses were English and literature classes. She lamented spending her hard-earned money on classes offered for free during high school, except policy forbade her and mandated that she instead take the test remediation courses. Heather no longer had any idea what career she might pursue, but she was keenly determined to earn a four-year degree.

Heather enjoyed going with me to Indian cultural events. Dr. Soni was one of the key organizers. Unlike the quiet persona that Dr. Soni portrayed at the pediatrics office, he was a talkative extrovert at such events. He founded BIMDA (Brevard Indo-American Medical and Dental Association) with one of his friends. First the group met in a garage, but it blossomed into elaborate affairs with semi-annual extravaganzas at the local Hilton.

"I told them to make you a member," Dr. Soni said to me.

"But your friends forbade it," I replied, "because I am neither a physician nor from India. Though they did grant permission for Jim and me to attend as guests."

At the weekend BIMDA continuing education conference, local physicians and dentists of Indian descent showcased medical products, attended lectures, debated hospital and national policies with old and new friends. Outdoors, caterers slapped flatbread dough onto the inside wall of a clay *tandoor* grill. Large foil trays of *samosas* beckoned hungry people to eat the fried-dough stuffed with potatoes, peas, onions, and chilies and dipped in tamarind or chili chutney.

Flamboyant entertainment preceded the evening's formal dinner. Afterward Dr. Soni announced music and dancing. Then, like the retelling of a favorite story, to everyone's amusement, Soni would sing sweet songs in Hindi to his wife to coax her to the dance floor. Rita Soni always playfully resisted.

On the surface, communication between our cultures may seem easy, but concepts of polite communication diverge greatly. Unrecognized offenses sometimes erupted in silent earthquakes. Neither Dr. Soni nor I knew how to avoid such misunderstandings or how to correct them, so we moved forward in what we did best, caring for our patients.

At the hospital, a male Indian colleague joined Dr. Soni and me as we proceeded along a corridor. Out of deference to their culture, I took several steps backward, eliminating myself from the circle of conversation. I nodded at Dr. Soni. "I'll head on to the nursery," I said quietly.

The skin of the newest born infant was a funny pink. Dr. Soni had already ordered a three-dimensional echocardiogram of the baby's heart with an arch view. A sonographer gobbed on warmed transducing gel. Inaudible ultrasonic sound waves echoed off the baby's heart, producing images of its beating chambers and moving valves.

Varying shades of colors portrayed the velocity, turbulence, and directional flow of blood along with any structural abnormality. If someone was actually peering directly at a beating heart, the preceding information would be impossible to discern. For interpretation, final images and measurements were transmitted via computer to Dr. Carson, a pediatric cardiologist in Orlando.

Having gone undetected on the mother's prenatal ultrasounds, Dr. Carson soon called with the devastating diagnosis—hypoplastic left ventricle, the same malformation that had ended Kyle's life. An ambulance transported the infant to Arnold Palmer Hospital for Children. Stabilizing medicines sustained the baby's life for a few days until a cardiac surgeon could perform a Norwood palliation, the first of three staged corrective surgeries.

Two months later, the mother brought the baby to the office for his vaccines. I cautioned her to have him checked any time he appeared ill. "Be especially careful with vomiting or diarrhea. It can disturb the delicate fluid balance that keeps his heart capable of pumping oxygenated blood to his brain," I warned.

"He breathes too fast, but it's normal for his cardiac condition." I pulsed my fingers in rhythm with the rapid, shallow movements of his chest. "Very subtle changes suggest worsening heart failure, such as feeding slower on the bottle, breathing faster, fingers and toes feeling colder, or appearing more quiet, pink, or blue. Call me anytime day or night, by my beeper or cell phone." I wrote down my numbers.

I saw the baby again at the end of summer. The baby had undergone the second surgery and was nine months old. He was happy, robust, and sat by himself without toppling. His mother said that his being a survivor caused great confusion.

"The ER doctor didn't believe the diagnosis. He refuted the idea that any baby could survive a hypoplastic left ventricle, even with surgery," she said.

I wrote a confirmation of the diagnosis on my prescription pad and signed it. From a pediatric cardiac surgery textbook, I made copies of the pages that had illustrations of the surgical procedures that he'd undergone and detailed treatment considerations and gave them to her. That year in Illinois gave me confidence about providing the baby's care.

CHAPTER 29]
DOSTANA
(FRIENDSHIP)

Two hundred dollars. Jamie's boyfriend, Marcus Barry, bid as he simultaneously shot up his hand.

"I recorded your pledge for posterity," Heather quipped. Marcus was a financially strapped college student.

"You really have to pay that," Jamie whispered, loud enough for those close-by to hear. She looked especially pretty in her evening gown.

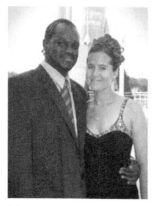

Marcus Barry and Jamie Giganti

The treasurer applauded Marcus's generosity in supporting the initiative. A middle-aged man proposed teaching people living in remote villages in India how to grow small plots of medicinal plants for their personal use as they lacked any access to medical care.

At Ma Krupa's annual fundraiser, Heather snapped photos as speakers pitched their projects to garner donations. Heather has a sharp, intuitive perception for photography. It seems a happy spin-off from when she was a confined and motionless baby. Back then, her seemingly vacant eyes must have actually been studying all she saw.

One of her first photos was a black and white of a nurse's smooth, manicured hand soothing an elderly patient's wrinkled one. Hospice selected it for their brochure's cover shot.

In her first year of college, Heather enrolled in photography and film courses. She became designated video photographer for several Indian festivals.

For a school project, Heather filmed a two-day cultural event and condensed it into a thirty-minute DVD. Slash-pine boughs arched over the "Welcome to India Fest" sign at Wickham Park. A poster featured Gandhi wearing round, Windsor-style glasses and homespun white *dhoti*. Heather positioned her tripod near the stage and held her ground when those jockeying for a better position tried to push her aside. I sat down on a nearby bench.

A local girl rendered an eloquent singing of "The Star-Spangled Banner." The Indian national anthem followed. On stage the regional dances began, resembling a living kaleidoscope. Performing Indian women were clad in brilliant saris and *choli* skirts—pink, turquoise, orange, yellow, greens, and golds, shimmering and exquisite. They adorned themselves with dozens of bangles on their wrists, dangling earrings, and ornate jewels in their hair. Men wore woven cotton tunic tops of brassy hues and muted colors. On their forehead, halfway between the eyebrows, a symbolic red *bindi* dot marked *ajna*, the seat of concealed wisdom.

The dancers' precise and graceful arm motions told stories of conflict, victory, love, and jubilance. Teenage girls teased young men with choreographed flirtation. As dusk fell, strobe lights focused on the stage now steeped in artificial fog. A finale commenced as fabulous as portrayed in actual Bollywood musicals. It formally closed the event, leaving the spectators wishing for more.

The India Fest chairman complimented Heather on the succinct video that she produced. "We are showing it at our next dinner. Your keen eyes captured all the important details," she said.

In 2006, for the first time since 1932, the American Academy of Otolaryngology, Head and Neck Surgery converged for their yearly conference outside of the United States. Heather jumped at the chance to visit Canada. She liked anything that involved travel and eating. Otolaryngologists flew in from North and South America, Europe, Asia, Africa, and Australia.

On September 17, Heather and I boarded a Delta flight out of Orlando and landed in Toronto at 10:00 a.m. An airport placard cautioned passengers to only accept rides at designated transportation counters, but we didn't see it. After we collected our suitcases and began contemplating what to do next, a man offered a taxi for fifty dollars. Exhausted, I impulsively agreed.

On the drive to the hotel, he recited a litany of tourist trivia, then turned down warehouse alley. "Faster this way," he said. He handed me a calendar, to write down departure information for our return to the airport. All the pages were blank. At that moment, I became acutely aware of an observation that I had discounted.

There was no company name painted on the cab, nor was there a taxi light on the roof. I called Jim from my cell phone, relaying who we were with, trying to sound confident. Fortunately the remaining miles proceeded uneventfully. The driver dropped us at the hotel entrance and offloaded our suitcases. I tipped him ten dollars.

"Spooky, when I opened that blank date book. So stupid of me," I said to Heather. "Maybe he isn't licensed, no bad motives. Look at this worn business card." The man had crossed out the bold-printed cab company ad and penciled in his personal name and phone number.

"Nothing happened, but cancel the reservation with that guy," Heather surmised. "Aren't you hungry?"

We checked into our hotel, and then strolled down a nearby sidewalk. International restaurants sat nearly on top of each other. A man wearing a turban stepped through his establishment's front doorway. "Come in," he invited. "Food very good." He escorted us past candlelit tables and extolled the deliciousness of the assorted dishes of the fragrant buffet. Heather and I ate our fill of spicy fare à la Punjab.

Afterward we dawdled and enjoyed looking at the intriguing lines of the high-rise architecture. Heather loaded black-and-white film into her camera and snapped some pictures. Once home, she'd develop the images in her college's darkroom.

"Excuse me, have we passed the Metro Toronto Convention Center?" I asked a passerby.

"It's up the road," he replied and motioned us onward. We headed that way, but did not find the entrance. Again I inquired, and received more detailed directions, but they seemed only to lead us toward assorted shops.

"Follow that left walkway," a young businessman advised. But we did not find any suggestion of a convention center. With frustrated puzzlement, we abandoned Front Street and took a tangent along the harbor. At last we deciphered our navigation problem; we couldn't see the forest for the trees so to speak.

Ordinary businesses with glass display windows formed much of the convention center's perimeter. The enormous facility occupied several blocks. Circuitously we were unaware that for several hours, we'd been meandering along its three sides that had unmarked secondary entry points. Only the main entrance road posted significant signage, which we finally stumbled upon.

Heather and I joined other conference attendees and collected our registration packets. An African otolaryngologist chatted with us. There was a shortage of ear, nose, and throat surgeons in her country. Intrigued with Heather's stream-lined audiology studies, the lady surgeon jotted down her e-mail address and requested that Heather send her information on the CPOP program.

"I'd be delighted," Heather replied, then started laughing as she recounted how it had taken us longer to find the convention center than to fly from Florida to Canada.

Now nineteen years old, Heather attended all the general sessions with me and a few select classes. During breaks, we introduced ourselves to whoever was nearby. They were always intrigued by Heather. "Keep writing about your daughter every chance you get. Miraculous stories help keep us motivated as a specialty," a California doctor encouraged me.

On a bus arranged by the Academy for family members, Heather took a day off from the meeting and toured the city. A couple of middle-aged women, who had travelled from China with their otolaryngologist husbands, befriended Heather. Late that afternoon, the three of them enjoyed a drenching at Niagara Falls.

Early in the evening while walking back to the hotel, Heather and I noticed a line of people so long that it wrapped around a city block. Curious, we jumped into last place and followed along until we discovered the reason for their patience. Reaching the event window at Rogers Centre stadium, we purchased the cheapest tickets available, five dollars each, for the Yankees-Blue Jays baseball game. Way, way up, we climbed the stairs and sat in the "500" seats situated behind the catcher.

The view thrilled us.

In the seventh inning, Yankees' Derek Jeter hit a two-run homer.

"How come the crowd is booing?" I asked Heather.

"We are in Toronto, Mom."

"Oh, yeah."

Soon after returning from Toronto, Jim and Heather took off to Philadelphia for her hands-on training in performing hearing tests. They stayed at the Hyatt, Penn's Landing on the Delaware River, which was where the three-day course was being held. Economy style, they'd brought along some canned goods; but discovered there was no microwave.

"There is a coffeepot," Heather suggested. Jim dumped in the Ravioli.

Cold, so cold outside, but they weren't prepared. Shivering, they tooled around town. Long rows of people blocked any chance to take photos of the Liberty Bell. They made sure to indulge in an authentic Philly Cheese Steak sandwich.

At the teaching stations, Heather practiced the use of tuning forks, an otoscope, a tympanometer, an otoacoustic emissions probe, and audiometers. "So much information, it is fascinating and almost overwhelming," Heather told me over the phone. "Masking is difficult. When testing a bad ear, the hearing of the good one is blocked with white noise so you don't crossover test the healthy one instead of the deaf one," she said.

On the last day, Heather scored a 100 percent on both the written and hands-on using the equipment exams.

Aunt Netty exclaimed an exuberant congratulations when she learned of Heather's perfect scores. She added an opinion on the state's standardized testing, "Abolish the FCAT; what does it know?"

To complete the CPOP certification requirements, Heather performed sixty of each of the following hearing tests: bone-and-air conduction tests with and without masking, and speech recognition evaluation. She did them under the direct tutelage of an audiologist and otolaryngologist (who happened to be her Uncle Mike). Sweet for her, and sweet for him.

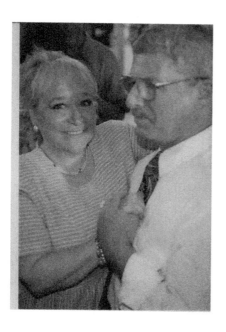

Celeste and Mark Hoffenberg

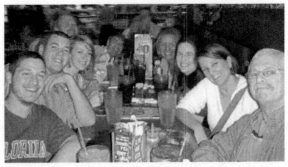

Heather and Valwood friends, always there for us

Of the original Valwood friends, there came the first wedding. Celeste and Mark's beautiful Haley was marrying her high-school soul mate, Josh. Handsome in dark tuxedos and maroon satin vests, proud father Mark and brother Nicholas greeted guests as they entered the church. Soft traditional music played.

"Heather is all grown up! Jamie, look at pretty you." Celeste exclaimed. Her health had taken a grievous downturn about the same time that Jim was diagnosed with cancer. The ceremony was her first excursion into the public in years.

Mark interrupted softly, "The wedding cake isn't here and the baker isn't answering her phone."

Celeste ignored him and kept talking to Heather. "I've become the way you once were," she said. A severe illness had catapulted her into the counter-world of Heather's previous sickly domain. A stint on a ventilator, lung damage rendered my dear friend barely able to walk or converse. How ironic, Celeste now leashed to an oxygen bottle. Still, her radiant beauty was only outshone by the bride. Her good soul and humor overshadowed all decline of her physical self.

Queen of festivities, elegant in a floral gown, Celeste rose up from her motorized chair. With sheer determination, she walked up the aisle with Nicholas at her side.

Proud father Mark beamed as he gazed on Haley, beautiful in her floor-length dress with train flowing behind. He lightly took hold of his daughter's arm and escorted her to the soon-to-be husband. A three-tiered lace veil gave an illusion that the top of Haley's head actually reached the groom's shoulder. Love radiated from the couple as they stood before the minister and exchanged their vows.

As one of the bridesmaids, Stephanie Little was in the receiving line. Squealing with delight she caught hold of her fiancé's elbow at the sight of Heather. "This is the miracle girl I told you about," she said. "I'm so happy and surprised to see you! We had lots of good times at the Gigantis. A half-dozen of us would climb into their hammock and swing."

I reminisced about her little brother. "Three years old, bouncing down the street like Tigger, but talking like a polished businessman and wearing a collared knit shirt. He'd extended his hand in a proper greeting. 'I'm Christopher John Little, and I'm looking for a new friend.'"

All evening, the exuberant newlyweds bebopped and rock-n-rolled. Both were talented musicians. In high school, Haley led the band as drum majorette when they marched in Macy's Thanksgiving Day Parade. She giggled almost nonstop as she danced with her handsome husband. They made the rounds, visiting each table. "Are you having fun?" she'd ask.

Magically the missing cake appeared. The caterer's van had broken down, but she borrowed a ride. Out front a limousine waited. The newlyweds ducked as they skipped out under the ceremonious tossing of birdseed as their guests bade them farewell.

Later that year, we traveled to Jacksonville for Stephanie and Sean's wedding. Haley graced the affair as one of the bridesmaids. At a stately waterfront venue with old brickwork and colorful floral arrangements, we sat with Mark and Nicholas at a round, linen-covered table. Unfortunately, Celeste was too ill to attend.

"Holy cow, is that Jamie?" Christopher John Little exclaimed, and he invited her to dance. He twirled her around the floor the way Popeye did with Olive Oyl in the animated cartoon.

Bruce and Barbara Maddern met us for Sunday breakfast. We shared vacation photo albums and updates on our children's activities. Heather chatted on about her life, but felt pressed to look over her audiology text book in preparation for performing for the next morning's audiogram. Scanning the review questions, Heather burst out laughing. "I know the answer to this one without looking it up—cholesteotoma."

Dr. Bruce reminded Heather to have her own hearing tested, to determine if there'd been any decline. Often the growths recur and claim both ears.

CHAPTER 30] SPACE EXTRAVAGANZA

Ed Mitchell, Apollo astronaut, tried to scientifically define the mysterious unspoken communication that led us to meet Heather.

President John F. Kennedy and his wife Jacqueline lost a baby to an early birth, a few months prior to the president's assassination. Born five and one-half weeks early on August 7, 1963 at a fairly robust 4 pounds ten and one-half ounces. Patrick Bouvier lived only thirty-nine hours, despite having the finest doctors in the country trying to save him. He died of the respiratory distress that affects premature babies.

Electrically powered ventilators were not yet developed, nor were neonatal intensive care units. I am remiss in that I have not devoted many words to the neonatologists that are dedicated to the health of tiny babies. Mostly because I never worked in a NICU more than an isolated day or two.

Dr. Sylvan Stool gave credit for the specialty's successes to the technology that was developed for the space program. It is intriguing that President Kennedy's commitment to land men on the moon brought that about.

The whimsy and dreams of the amazing space program created an imaginative backdrop to all years in the life of my family. Dad encouraged the grandchildren to pursue engineering by kindling their interest without being pushy. Until the Challenger disaster, Jamie's ambition was to become a veterinarian caring for animals on space missions.

My dad had obtained a car pass for viewing an evening launch of the Space Shuttle Discovery from pad 39B. Jim, Heather, and I went with him. We rode through the Center's checkpoint and parked on two-lane NASA Causeway, flanked on both sides by the Banana River. Spotlights illuminated the distant launch pad. Security restrictions rendered the river empty of boats and the sky devoid of planes.

To claim a spot among the crowd lounging together like seals on a beach, we spread a blanket over trampled-down grass. A man and his son wrestled jovially while the mother read her novel, ignoring them. No coolers were anywhere; none allowed since the September 11 disaster. Powerful mailbox-sized cameras rested on tripods near the water's edge. Personal cameras outnumbered binoculars ten to one. Behind us on the roadway sat a staggering line of empty busses.

STS-116's mission was to bring supplies and a truss to the International Space Station and rewire its power-supply system. "Attention!" the announcer broadcast over loudspeakers. "Please stay out of the river, and be wary of our local residents—alligators. In the unlikely occurrence of a mishap at Complex 39, vapors or a toxic cloud could pour into the viewing area. In that event, immediately proceed to your vehicle and listen for further instructions."

International voices melded into a background buzz. A generator powering a cooking tent produced a deafening drone. "Burgers, hot burgers," touted the chef.

"I'm hungry," Heather said.

"Tell the cook how you like it," Jim said.

"Well done. Catsup, mustard, pickle, onions, and mayo please," Heather requested.

"Anyone else?" Jim asked, and pulled out his wallet.

In the darkness, the launch pad emitted a soft white glow. Excitement perked. Countdown to blast off. At T-minus six seconds, four-hundred thousand gallons of water began dumping on launch pad 39B. As the engines flamed, massive clouds of steam erupted, dampening sound waves that would otherwise damage the pad and the Shuttle and shatter windows up to twenty-five miles away.

Fiery light from burning rocket fuel danced onto drifting, white and fluffy clouds, dusting them with iridescent colors. Roosting island birds rose skyward, not in a panic, but in a silent V-formation. The explosion of flames and sounds with crescendos of palpable ground-shaking vibrations united the awed viewers, who burst into an accolade of spontaneous cheers. All gazed upward at the rocket's rapid ascent. It's shrinking, flickering glow flared momentarily.

"Is something wrong?" Heather asked.

"That was the successful separation of the solid rocket boosters," Granddad explained. Two glowing embers tumbled toward earth.

Relieved, we kept sight of the spark that was the Shuttle as it thrust onward, growing smaller. Its vapor trail expanded, lengthened, and wrapped around itself. Sound reverberation ceased. The birds returned, still flying in formation to take their repose on the nearby island.

"Awesome! It was stupendous, Granddad," Heather exclaimed.

Thanksgiving. Candles flickered on the festive dinner tables. Coffee dripped through the brewer. Nineteen-year-old Heather cut me a slice of pie and spoke in a whisper. "I think something's wrong with Granddad Fritz. He kept spilling cherries on his chin." I too had noticed, but suppressed any contemplation on its significance. "Geeze," Heather commented, straight to the point. "We're going to lose Dad, and now Granddad is dying too."

One month later, doctors diagnosed an inoperable brainstem tumor. Nothing dampened his good nature and enthusiasm. Dad required assistance twenty-four hours a day.

Weekdays, he resided at my brother's or sister's house. On weekends, Jim, Heather, or I stayed with him in his home. His mouth numbness increased. He could no longer eat fried chicken because he couldn't tell the difference between meat and bone. At meals a bib protected his clothes from tidbits of food that spilled from his mouth.

"Sorry," he apologized.

"I don't care," Heather reassured him.

"I do," he replied with emphasis unusual for him.

"Want to play Rummy Cube, Granddad? I'll win."

"I beat you last time. I'll do it again," he replied, chuckling.

Each weekend, Dad would tell his favorite space stories, and I recorded them. On his paperwork table, I happened upon letters he'd penned in shaky handwriting to his astronaut friends. "We're celebrating my daughter's fiftieth birthday at the Astronaut Hall of Fame Induction Gala. Look for me; I'm the old man in the wheelchair with a pirate patch over one eye."

Dad covered his left eye to prevent double vision, because it no longer lined up with the right. Once, Dad used the nuisance to his advantage. At an Indian event, the belly dancer dazzled all with her veil, scarves, sparkling jangles and costume of embroidered chartreuse. Her fluid movements mesmerized even the musicians. I watched them watching her. My father tapped my shoulder and grinned.

"She is my therapy. I removed the patch so I could see two of her."

For the upcoming summer, Dad wanted a grand family reunion as it would be his last. He rented a vacation house in Key Largo. In preparation, we practiced snorkeling. Heather steadied him on the pool stop while I assisted him with flippers, mask, and snorkel. Diving forward, he metamorphosed into a healthier man and swam strong laps.

I treaded water, keeping watch on his bald head moving through the surface as it began to submerge. I'd grip his life vest to lift him higher.

"I was fine until you came over," he protested.

"No you weren't. Your snorkel was about to dip under the water. Try tilting your noggin more forward."

Out of the pool and toweled off, Heather would guide Dad and his walker indoors to the living room. She lavished an abundance of care, same as he had always given her.

At work, Becky and I proposed a hundred preposterous ways to get my Dad out of the boat and into the water—sling shot, diving board, or towed on an inflatable raft. Nah, he'd be shark bait. In slapstick absurdity, we continued the nonsense, though intense seriousness weighted the underlying question.

"I'll mount a playground slide onto the boat. Granddad can slip into the ocean," I remarked to Tony.

"The boat would look stupid," Tony replied.

"Just joking. How would he climb back on board?" Expensive electronic water lifts were out of the question. The solution. A welder installed a wide platform off the stern and added extra rungs to its underwater ladder. He fashioned removable hand-grips that extended four feet above the upper gunwales, so Dad wouldn't have to stoop.

Friday morning, I reminded the office staff to stop the schedule at 2:00 p.m. "I'll order pizza so we can work through lunch and lock up early."

"Dr. Soni's time is blocked too. Why?" Tiffany asked me, looking puzzled.

"For my birthday," I replied.

"Oh yeah," she said. I wished all the staff could have attended the Space Center gala, but it was too expensive.

All phone calls returned, I was heading out when a woman knocked at the office's locked back door. Her ten-year-old son was wheezing. "Okay, but no more, otherwise my family will miss everything," I said, and quickly tended to the child.

Hurry, hurry, hurry. At home I showered. Jamie, Heather, and I slipped on loosely fitted blouses to keep from messing up our soon-to-be fancy hair. Evening gowns, high heels, and jewelry were readied the night before.

Off to our hair-styling appointments at a salon with a prestigious name and close to home.

"Mom, how much will it cost?" Jamie asked.

"I forgot to inquire."

"Shouldn't we ask the price?" she persisted.

"Too late now; we want to be gorgeous, don't we?" I answered.

A chic young woman confirmed our appointments. Jamie whispered in my ear. "The salon seems really expensive; ask how many dollars. We can leave."

There were no other customers. Due to our narrow-time constraint, the shop scheduled it that way. One-on-one spoiling commenced. Each beautician sparkled a colorful, quirky personality. Like long-lost friends, the six of us jabbered and gushed in full mirth as the stylists twisted, pulled, and sprayed our hair into works of art. Heather looked stunning with a modern, upward Asian spike;

Jamie belonged in a princess's castle with her long ringlets upswept into an intricate pattern and bedecked with flowers and jewels. I felt elegant with soft flowing waves and woven curls, secured with at least one hundred hidden bobby pins.

Then the bill, and suppressed shock: $350. I tried to act cool.

We pulled up to the house at the same time that Marcus did. His friend spent three hours weaving Marcus's hair into handsome cornrows. "Mom, who looks the best? Me or Jamie?" Marcus asked, his eyes shining with affection for my daughter. "Pick me, pick me, me, me," Marcus teased. He laughed the rich, captivating laugh of his family—begotten of Anguilla and St. Maarten, French and Dutch sweetened into one.

"Hmmm, hard decision, let me think. Fabulous, but," I glanced over at my Jim, dressed to impress. "I choose an Italian husband. He's the Ritz."

"Hey, I thought I was most beautiful," Grandma Jean (Jim's mom) objected.

Hurry, hurry, hurry. Only ten minutes to change into our formal attire and leave in the van. Heather hoped to meet Space Shuttle astronaut Steve Oswald, who had once autographed an eight-by-ten photograph for Granddad to give to us. He'd relished learning about the miracle of Heather. "Enjoyed working with Fritz . . . hearing all the stories of his grandkids and trips to Jacksonville."

All were rendezvousing at Dad's house before departing for the Kennedy Space Center Visitor Complex. Dad owned a tuxedo; but not wanting to outdo his guests, he wore a classic dark suit and tie. With great chivalry, Jim pinned a boutonnière to Dad's lapel and presented me with a rose corsage, a preamble to a night of living the stuff of fairy tales.

Jamie sashayed around, distributing seating charts for the thirty guests sitting at three tables of ten. To the left of Dad, Jim and I would sit; and to his right would be Mahesh and Rita Soni. "If I keep them close, I'll have an opportunity to introduce them to the astronauts," Dad said.

After passing through security searches, we mingled in the welcoming reception, sipping wine and sampling hors d'oeuvres. Tour buses took us to the main event at the Apollo/Saturn V Center. Nineteen outstanding science and engineering college students would be recognized for their accomplishments, and each awarded a $10,000 scholarship.

Inside the Center, at least fifty servers dressed in black and white stood along a wall, biding time until dinner. Overhead, affixed to the ceiling of the huge hall, the enormous Saturn V moon rocket loomed majestically. Its five F1 thrusters are the most powerful single-nozzle liquid fueled engines ever flown. Around the corner, a display of the lunar module and rover gleamed with understated magnificence.

As a child, Dad's key role in the moon landings seemed part of the family's ordinary routine. Cooking dinner for the Apollo astronauts at our house seemed special, yet part of the usual fabric of life. Meeting them again as an adult is an extraordinary honor. All conversations with astronauts are memorable, but two stand out because they also spoke of the divine.

I was fourteen years old when I first met Ed Mitchell. He was sitting next to my parents on their green velvet couch. It was 1972. The year before, he'd piloted the lunar module for Apollo 14, landing it on the Fra Mauro formation. Walking the new frontier of the moon's surface propelled him not only on a pondering of outer space, but of inner spiritual space as well.

Sitting on that couch, in his hand, he held a misshapen ring— bent with psychic mind energy. He mesmerized me with its story and the one of how he'd taken his mother, who had been stricken with sudden blindness, to a Tibetan Buddhist healer. The mystic meditated, prayed a mantra, and swept his hands over the woman's eyes, restoring her vision. Though later on, she dwelt on what she considered a thorn to her sense of propriety (the man was not Christian), and her blindness recurred.

At the gala, when I recalled meeting him as a teenager, Ed Mitchell's face lit up. Matters of faith had led each of us to the spirituality of India. He explained further, "On the return from the moon, gazing at the blue sphere of planet Earth and the vastness of the stars, I experienced a Wow! Eureka! A feeling that all molecules, mine and space, were interconnected. What kind of mind created such a feeling?" he said. Digging through the ancient Sanskrit Hindi writings, he discovered a description of the experience and its name, *Samadhi*.

Subsequently, Ed Mitchell dedicated his energy to the study of psychic events, intuition, and consciousness as explainable phenomena bridging science, mysticism, and physics. "Nonlocal quantum holograms," he said. "Research is proving that objects or beings emit packets of information on their structure and existence. A summation of life experiences can be transported as a wave length without constraint as to time and place and can be viewed by another."

"That could explain prayer?" I asked.

"Prayer goes out there as energy to the universe," he replied in the affirmative.

"And meditation quiets the mind to receive an answer," I said.

Charlie Duke, lunar module pilot for Apollo 16, viewed space as an intellectual experience. Spirituality came years later. He was the tenth man to walk on the moon and drove the lunar rover over its rough terrain. He stressed that launch requires the successful interplay of many thousands of parts.

"Take-off felt as if it were shaking us to pieces. The feeling of this astronaut was 'I just had to keep holding on.' Fuel burned, creating a crushing G-force of 4.5 times our weight on earth.

Wham! The first stage shut down so violently I thought we'd blown up. It separated, and the rocket rode smoothly. It was perfect. Windows then unveiled a view of Earth, an incredible sight. Two and a half hours later we accelerated to almost twenty-six thousand miles per hour, and we were on our way."

Praying for a stronger marriage was when he and his wife found God. "I developed an insatiable desire to read the Bible and began listening with my heart, not my mind, and put it into practice. We were restored in joy and love. There was no angelic music, but a sure knowledge of peace began to come." Anyone who makes their acquaintance feels the glow of their spirituality.

Throughout the celebration of Astronaut Gala 2007, the atmosphere swirled with the best of faith, culture, and intellect woven together into magnificent dreams of the past, present, and future. Master of ceremonies, Apollo 15's Al Worden, suggested that all find their seats so he could begin the formal introductions of the astronauts. As he spoke, each courageous space man strode in one-at-a-time from alternating sides of the room. Hushed in wonder, we watched the magnificent rocket men.

"John Glenn," Mahesh whispered in awe as the national hero and his wife, Annie, passed within ten feet. All attendees rose in respect and delivered a thunderous standing ovation. In 1962, John Glenn was the first American to orbit the earth. At age seventy-seven, he accomplished another amazing first and became the oldest person to fly on a Space Shuttle mission. In addition, he served the country as a senator from Ohio for twenty-five years.

"Remember when we spoke with them at another fundraiser?" Dad asked.

"Impossible to forget. They are warm and eloquent and have a marvelous aura," I answered.

All in all, thirty-five astronauts strode past us. Many of them stopped for a significant pause and greeted my father as their most revered guest.

Next, Al Worden introduced Shuttle astronauts, Michael Coats, Steven Hawley, and Jeffrey Hoffman, who were being inducted into the Hall of Fame. Video clips portrayed highlights of their careers, after which they spoke for themselves.

Heather pushed Dad in his wheelchair over to where Fred Haise of Apollo 13 was sitting. "Fred and I collaborated on the initial testing of Lunar Module 3 for its maiden flight. We would conduct unofficial dry runs," Dad said. "Moon travel had never been tried before. All of the nation's prestige depended on its success." In formal testing, the astronauts would suit up under depressurized conditions. Any error or warning light would abort the procedures and postpone further testing to a later day, which would consequently push back the possibility of America's first footstep on the moon.

"Fred and I smoothed out the process prior to the official testing," Dad said. "Fred would sit in the simulator, or mock-up, and I'd read him the procedure."

"I'd repeat it back word for word and execute the instructions," Haise said. "Any deviations or abnormalities, we'd troubleshoot and revise the written procedure until we got it right. We marked all the newly instituted changes on the official protocol. In the original writing, there were things you'd forget to take into account," Fred Haise said. "A lit-up warning light could take a lot of investigative time. Sometimes after studying it, we'd conclude nothing was wrong, 'Ah, that light is supposed to go on.'"

"Emulating how equipment functions in a lunar environment is hard to achieve," Fred Haise emphasized. "Designed for one-sixth gravity, the lunar module's construction material is flimsy on Earth. If not careful, your hand could push through it. Fans specially designed for use on the moon would burn up if utilized on Earth."

We didn't want the festivity to end, but of course it did. Space Center tour buses returned all guests to the Visitor's Center. Instead of being stuck in the sluggish departing traffic jam, our ensemble loitered in the parking lot. Talented family members improvised the pavement as an impromptu stage, and the entertainment began.

Marcus flipped into a single-handed hand stand, initiating a series of the dance-like moves of the Capoeira, an Afro-Brazilian martial art. John Widick removed his jacket and began sparring with Marcus using a fluid leg sweep.

Doug strummed the guitar and serenaded us with some popular songs. He and John had brought their *tablas* (Indian drums), hoping to play ragas with Dr. Soni, but time ran short. I was very disappointed.

"It is okay, Ann," Dr. Soni said. "We have a long future."

The traffic thinned, and we departed to gather at my childhood home. Mom lit fifty birthday candles. We relished eating moist carrot cake and abundant frosting, relaxing on the couches or carpeted floor. Conversation was witty and spilling over with silliness, but we were too worn out to jump in the pool and play Marco, Polo. It was a very fine night, stupendous!

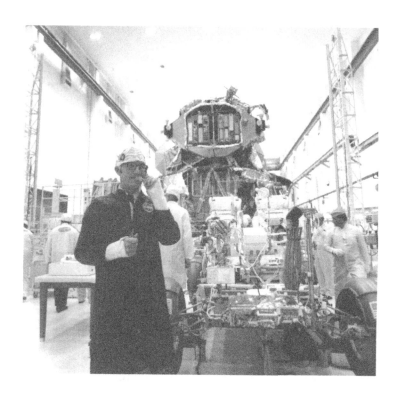

Granddad Fritz Widick, chief test conducter for lunar module, broke both wrists playing softball against the astronauts, running into home base.

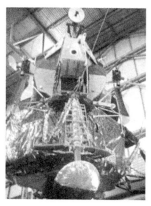

CHAPTER 31] FULL CIRCLE

Fortune had it that Jim was enjoying a partial remission from the leukemia and lymphoma. "How much longer until we leave for Key Largo?" Dad asked. Fatigued and edgy from packing, Jim and I had more preparation to do.

"I'm all ready. I can drive Granddad Fritz. We'll get there fast," Heather offered. She loaded his medical gear, and we stuffed the van with boxes of groceries. Time had brought them full circle. Granddad and granddaughter, caretaking roles now reversed, zoomed off on our annual pilgrimage to the island of no cares.

Arriving at the rental paradise, Heather maneuvered their vehicle in backwards to hasten the offloading of provisions. Accidentally she pushed on the gas pedal, instead of the brake and accelerated into the driveway's chain-link fence. Granddad wobbled around with the aid of his walker. "The van is intact. You mangled the gate a little bit," he told her.

Heather phoned of their safe arrival, extolling the virtues of the house, not mentioning the damaged gate. "It's painted a lemon yellow. Outside by the canal, it has a thatched-roof gazebo and a barbeque grill. The view of the Atlantic Ocean is awesome!"

Jim and I didn't leave until early the next morning. Towing the boat lengthened the travel time. In Homestead, we stopped to fuel the car and boat and take a quick detour toward the Everglades. The "Robert Is Here" fruit stand has been selling scrumptious shakes for over fifty years. Scoops of rich ice cream and freshly picked sun-ripened fruit are blended in tall, old-fashioned metal canisters until frosted. When our tantalizing order was ready, they'd notify us over ramshackle speakers.

Meanwhile, we meandered through the wooden bins of kiwis, papayas, and watermelons, and then strolled past squawking parrots to the farm animals. A footpath circled around billy goats, giant tortoises, and strutting fat turkeys. Ducks swam in the watering hole. Reaching the end, we washed our hands in lever-pumped well water.

Sipping on our delicious, fruity milkshakes, we clambered back into the van and began traversing the barren eighteen-mile stretch of US 1 that ran through secluded waters and mangrove islands. Suddenly Jim shrieked, jerking back his shoulder. "A jumbo bumble bee flew in and landed on me!" Hollering his on-going distress, somehow Jim managed to keep the van and boat steady on the road.

"Relax. I'll shoo it out. Roll down both front windows and pop open the rest." Mom unlatched her seatbelt and moved forward.

Jim sounded an even greater alarm. "Yikes! The bee dropped into the seat of my pants. It is buzzing."

"I'm not reaching in there," Mom said.

We busted out into hilarious laughter, even Jim, though his mirth was intermixed with fearful yelps. Luck had the insect forsake its hideaway and float off on the breeze.

Arriving at vacation paradise, Jim and Tony drove to the ramp and launched our twenty-one foot boat. We named it *Triple Tales*, a play on words that referred to the fish species, the wagging tails of our three dogs, and the life story of each of our children.

Tony motored the boat through the canals, slowing as he neared the dock. Attired in our swimsuits, we climbed aboard. My dad wore a wetsuit for greater warmth. He sat down into the sturdy nautical chair that Tony had installed for his benefit. Seven miles offshore at Molasses Reef, we tethered to a mooring ball. Jim no longer swam, due to his precarious health. He'd watch over our safety from the vantage of the boat.

A frail, skinny old man, my dad balanced on the dive platform, contemplating his dilemma. "Do you think I can climb back into the boat?" he asked. We hadn't practiced, lest failure take its chance at creeping in.

"You'll succeed, Fritz," Jim affirmed. "Floating away on the deep blue sea like a giant jelly fish is not an option."

Wobbly, Dad maneuvered down the ladder and plunged in. Snorkeling restored his grace. He and I swam together for about an hour of reef exploration before tackling the get-back-into-the-boat hurdle. Dad ascended, conquering each ladder rung, one at a time—as determined as Heather had been so long ago climbing from the depths of Devil's Millhopper. Resting on the platform, he grasped the handgrips and hoisted his feet over the gunwale. Maneuvering the way to his seat, we cheered him sitting there, one with nature, tall and stoic.

A thunderstorm blew in while Tony steered up the canal to the house. The sky blackened. As we secured ropes to the dock cleats, wind gusts bent palm trees over until nearly parallel to the concrete seawall. Dad scrambled with his walker. We hurried inside, striding barefoot over sharp gravel.

"Whoops, forgot my hat." Tony dashed back to the boat and retrieved it.

Electric power in the neighborhood blacked out, triggering a loud clanging of the house's security system. The feature is designed to dissuade burglars from snipping an alarm's electrical source in an effort to silence it, as the opposite occurs. No reset instructions were found. Jim considered smashing the device. Several deafening hours of incessant noise ensued.

At last, a utility crew restored electricity. Peace resumed. The realtor returned our earlier desperate calls. She said a small tornado had skipped down the canal. Stuck in its calm center, we hadn't recognized how those folded-over palms resembled televised images of hurricane-force winds.

"Yo, Tony saved his hat from a twister," Heather teased.

"It's a nice hat," Tony countered.

A life-sized sculpted mermaid was mounted under the stairwell. Her curves were flesh color, and her tail was painted emerald. "She visits me at night. I find her scales in my bed when I waken," my dad said, chuckling at his own corny supposition.

"Granddad, I get paid to scuba dive and drive boats for a living, how lucky am I?" Jamie boasted. She had driven up from Marathon, where she worked for Florida Fish and Wildlife. An enthusiastic marine biologist, she conducted research on promoting the health of coral reefs and the tropical and sport fish populations.

Luck let her rent a rustic, waterfront duplex near the Seven Mile Bridge. Hurricane Wilma had scared away the previous renters. Its storm surge had sent waves over many rooftops. My dad asked Jamie if he could celebrate his seventy-sixth birthday at her duplex. Of course, she agreed.

His momentous weekend arrived, and we trekked back to the Keys. Even more frail, Dad slipped his arms through a life vest and snapped the clasps. Several fat iguanas sunned on the concrete walk that went around the side of the house to the postage-stamp sized backyard near the dock. Carefully clutching the boarding grips, Dad stepped over the gap between the seawall and the boat. Tony settled him into the special nautical chair.

"Have fun fishing," Jim said. He'd elected to stay behind and rest, then he and Jamie would shop for a birthday cake when she got off work.

We cruised around the bend and over shallow waters to the back country, not the ocean. Tony switched on the GPS and began motoring out to a secret, guaranteed-to-catch fish spot. Smooth bay waters were barely wrinkled.

"Ann?" Dad called. The boat traveled quietly in the calm water, yet I had to lower my ear toward Dad's whispery voice to hear him.

"My head is wobbling," Dad said.

"I can fix that," I said. I knelt behind him and gently positioned my hands to cradle the sides of his balding head and pressed my forearms alongside his neck and shoulders and onto the back of his chair, utilizing all muscles in my body to maintain a steadfast splint. Tony sped the boat onward over still waters. I felt peace and joy and the presence of God in the beauty of the backwaters and the diligent tending of my children, in Jim's ongoing struggle to survive.

"Hey, Ann." Dad interrupted my thoughts, his eyes twinkling. "Maybe we can design a head-stabilizing support that bolts to my chair, so you don't have to manually brace my neck from snapping. And so, even when the seas are rough, I can still go out in the boat."

"Pops, I'm sure you and Jim can figure out something. We'll do it."

A deeper reason I like the seas is that shades of aqua nothingness shut out the noise of the mind. That day, powder blue sky arched over flat turquoise waters. Other than a couple of small islands, nothing broke up the endless blue, no buildings or birds or boats. Nothing disrupted the calming silence, until the delight of seeing a turtle's head breach the water, a lone jellyfish, or circling high above a frigate bird whose silhouette resembled an elegant boomerang. Sighting a dozen or so diving birds signified fish feeding below and kindled thoughts of catching them.

We reached our fishing spot. Tony slowed the engine and shifted the gear into neutral. "Heather, drop the anchor, please."

Opening the front hatch, she lifted the anchor and ran her fingers along its line, checking that sound knots secured the anchor to its chain, the chain to the rope, and the rope to the boat's eyebolt. She fed the anchor under the bow rail and released it, careful not to entangle herself in the rapidly following line. Allowing for slack, she secured the rope around a cleat on the boat's bow.

Tony ran the engine in reverse to check if the anchor held. "Good job, Heather," he said, and toggled on the drift alert. Overboard went the chum bag into the water. Oils emitted from its thawing five-pound block of scrap-bait formed a lengthening slick that minnows and small fish would scavenge. Bigger fish would prey on the smaller fish, and with luck, the tastiest would strike at one of our hooks.

"Something's feeding back there," Tony said. Onto his hook he threaded a live shrimp and cast into the middle of the slick. "Yeah, I just got slammed!" Tip up, reeling, tip down, pump up, reeling, avoid slack. He played the fish until it came to the surface. Underneath I slipped a net and lifted, in case it spit the hook. Tony grasped his catch, then placed it on a ruler built into the top of the cooler.

"A nice mangrove snapper," Granddad Fritz complemented him.

"Thirteen inches. What's the limit?" Tony asked. Florida law penalizes anyone taking undersized species—as serious as a year in jail and maybe seizing your boat and car.

"The limit is twelve inches total length. Thirteen is good," Heather said.

Tony pulled in two more snappers. "These two-aught circle hooks are the shiznits," he said.

Heather began reeling in fast.

"You have a fish on?" Granddad asked.

"False alert," Heather replied. She baited her bare hook with a chunk of fresh-caught ballyhoo and wiped its slime on her shorts.

"Feeding the fish, Heathy?" Tony razzed her.

"Someone dropped a hook," I said.

"It is near the wall. You won't step on it," Tony answered.

"Hmm, how come I know it's there?" I retorted.

"Look at Mom's foot." Heather giggled. Drops of blood dripped from the fresh puncture near my small toe. Tony plucked up the nuisance.

A long shadow swirled by, its tail fin showing. "Dang shark is after my bait," I said.

"Catch it!" Tony exclaimed.

"I don't want to," I said.

Swishing its tail, the creature propelled its gaping jaws out of the water. I yanked back on my rod, flipping the bait out of its closing teeth. The fish circled wide and deep, becoming lost from view.

Tony was ready when the shadow returned. He drifted his line around to my side of the boat. I reeled to avoid catching the thing. Despite that, my fishing line flew out, the drag zinged. Tony's line zipped out simultaneously.

"I caught the dang shark!" I protested. "Whoops! I reeled in a fat snapper. You've got the shark, Tony." He muscled the fish in near to the boat. Heather grabbed the landing net.

"Not a shark; it is a cobia," Granddad proclaimed. In the water, its shape and swimming motion resembled a shark's, but it is leaner. To the fork of the tail, the cobia measured thirty-two inches—one inch shy of its limit. Tony threw it overboard.

"Mom yanked her bait out of a cobia's mouth," Heather said, breaking into more giggles. Looking toward the horizon, she pulled out her camera. "It's going to be an extra-sweet sunset."

Fleecy clouds drifted in front of the sun. Pink colors spewed forth that brightened to salmon. Puddles of blush spilled all over the blue sky. Nearing the horizon, the sun sent glowing tethers of light that melted to tangerine along the water line.

We kept fishing. Our catch included grouper, ladyfish, mackerel, the cobia, many snapper, and a young shark. Heather wrapped Granddad with a flannel blanket and covered his head with a warm, knit cap. The background darkness of the sky grew profound, so black that within it we would have disappeared. Instead the stars dazzled with supreme intensity and showered us in magical brightness, as we were anchored far away from any town or artificial light.

"Heather, look at the galaxies. Clusters of stars glowing in endless layers. This is a terrific birthday," Granddad said.

Back at Jamie's duplex, he opened a few gifts. We lit the candles, sang our well-wishes, and gratefully tumbled under our bedcovers.

Later that same month, Jim, Jamie, Grandma, Heather, and I flew to Washington, D.C. The Academy of Otolaryngology had selected a poster version of my graduate work, "Airway Suction: Not So Simple," for continuous display throughout their five-day 111th annual meeting. Out of submissions from all over the world, they'd only accepted two hundred research posters.

A security guard directed Heather and me to the great hallway after glancing at our identification badges. Mine had a flashy, distinguishing presenter's ribbon. Jim tagged along and assisted in setting up the poster.

Grandma Jean was eighty-something. The hotel doorman laughed at her complaints of sore feet. Jamie delighted in mapping out a strenuous tourist itinerary. Highlights included an energetic Little Richard street concert backdropped by the Smithsonian, touring the Holocaust museum, and watching jazz dancers perform at the Kennedy Center.

Dining at an Ethiopian restaurant raised some confusion. No forks or spoons. The waiter spooned mounds of aromatic concoctions on a circular sponge bread. We copied the other patrons and tore off pieces, dipped them into the tasty dishes, and consumed the dollops with our fingers.

Heather and I joined them most evenings. Boarding the subway, Grandma grabbed an overhead rung and stood fast. A tough-looking youth offered up his seat.

"I'm not too old to stand," Grandma objected, and rattled on, putting on airs of great offense. A young, deaf woman watched the exchange, not comprehending. Her beau interpreted in sign-language as the scene further unfolded. The deaf woman's concern broadened to a smile as she came to understand the gist of their conversation.

Next, a scruffy punk-rocker offered to relinquish his seat. Grandma responded with even more virulent indignation. Along came a third man, a flamboyant bow-tied gentleman. He too had his polite offer of seat-giving shot down by Grandma's sharp words.

Fancy Heather. Fancy me. We dressed elegantly for the Academy's formal dinner reception. Most of the pediatric otolaryngologists knew of Heather from the story in *Woman's Day*. Eager to meet Dr. Robin Cotton, the surgeon who had developed the laryngotracheoplasty procedure, we signed up for one of his courses. Hearing him teach seemed a dream. Afterward, I expressed great appreciation for his dedication. "Heather was three years old when she underwent the LTP surgery. We consider it miraculous and magical. It changed everything," I said.

"The quality of her voice sounds great," Dr. Cotton commented.

"A video of her trachea and its graft, taken when she had ear surgery as a teenager, shows that her airway has grown normally. No dimpling or scarring. No detecting which tissue had been the graft," I said.

"Heather, what studies are you pursuing in college?" Dr. Cotton asked.

"I am applying to attend nursing school," she answered.

"May you have success in all your endeavors," Dr. Cotton replied. They shook hands, and both broadened their smiles.

"Thanks again," Heather said.

Heather and I found it hard to walk away and let the moment end.

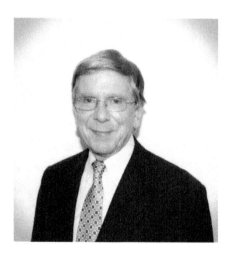

Dr. Robin Cotton, pediatric otolaryngologist, creator of the airway reconstructive procedure, laryngotracheoplasty

CHAPTER 32] ST. KITTS

B y the end of that same September, the one of taking my dad fishing and going to the Washington, DC conference, we buried my father. He lived in the amazing era of the dawn of space exploration. To his family, he championed our dreams and instilled confidence. We'll always miss him.

On a happier note, at the beach above the rolling waves, Matt heaped up a giant wall of damp sand. Into it, he etched out the letters I LOVE HEATHER. The affection in his heart bloomed larger than any symbol he could create. Heather and Matt first became friends when they worked together at McDonalds. They got reacquainted while Heather was working for my brother doing hearing tests. She happened to answer the phone when Matt called to schedule a tonsillectomy. "I know you," she said and thus their romance began.

As a younger man, Jim had thought good nutrition and exercise guaranteed health and living to an old age. We learned the folly of that thinking. Fortunately, Jamie, Tony, and Heather's vibrant steps toward independent adulthood cushioned the reality of Jim's decline.

Never free of disease, Jim's chronic leukemia and lymphoma simmered, sporadically erupting like a volcano; death always loitered in the shadows. We continued to rely on God, listening for his guidance anywhere he might speak, sometimes through prayer, the church, temple, family, friends, and often strangers, and the ever-present quiet guidance of the Holy Spirit.

Hoping for an improvement, Jim enrolled in a research cancer regimen on the west coast of Florida. For several months, one of our children or I drove him there three days a week. Ironically, on the study's drug protocol, Jim's lymphoma tumors grew larger, and fibrous scarring proliferated in his lungs. That ended the experiment.

To have more time to tend to Jim, I stopped working for Dr. Soni. Instead I began securing temporary travel assignments, contracting by the day or week. While at a six-week temp job for a pediatrician in Palmetto, Florida, Heather called me. Jim had spiked a 104-degree fever, and was stumbling and hallucinating.

"Call an ambulance," I said.

Infection from a scratched mosquito bite had poisoned his blood, put clots in his lungs, and set his kidneys to failing. During his week-long hospitalization, and for the umpteenth time, Heather updated me on his condition, labs, testing, and medications. At my job, I told no one about his illness. I could not take any days off work. Any concern about my reliability would slam the door to future travel assignments, not just at their office, but anywhere.

Jim rallied. Once he regained some strength, he set up a desk and computer station next to a sunny window in our family room. Florida Tech continued to provide him the flexibility to work partial days either from home or at the office, even with an intravenous needle in his arm. When working on-site at the university, a co-worker always ate lunch with him and encouraged him to eat. Most days his mom would pick him up for a midday meal and nap.

Life zipped forward to 2010 with the usual ups and downs. The backward blessing of Jim's illness is that we tried not to postpone what we might could enjoy each day. He avoided taking chemotherapy like the plague. As always if his condition greatly deteriorated, he'd take the oldest and safest chemo pill in order to survive to the next vacation, birth, wedding, or graduation.

Heather completed her basic college studies and wanted to transfer to a four-year university. She still aspired to a career in nursing. With the bad economy, chances were slim. Too many applicants vying for scant slots.

"Another rejection letter," Heather complained.

"Maybe change your dream job?"

"I could be an investigator, I watch crime shows," Heather replied.

"I thought you didn't like associating with criminals," I said.

"I don't," she answered.

"What sort of people do you think investigators pursue?" I asked.

"Oh yeah, not a good choice," she said.

An Internet search chanced upon the International University of Nursing. Its campus overlooked the ocean in the island country of St. Kitts, located in the Caribbean. The nursing school was situated on the same grounds as the medical school. The two schools shared modern classrooms and state-of-the-art teaching labs equipped with elaborate mannequins for learning examinations and procedures.

Heather's acceptance gifted her with a unique opportunity. While in St. Kitts, she would learn the basics of nursing and experience old-style health care under third-world conditions. To finish up, she'd transfer to a partner university in the United States.

Late summer, I dropped Heather at the Miami airport, feeling foolish. Hurricane Earl was barreling toward St. Kitts. Boyfriend Matt and sister Jamie arrived first. They'd keep Heather company for her first week of living in a foreign land.

Weather conditions deteriorated. Heather's plane was the last one permitted to land. Shopkeepers finished boarding up all stores. Scarce groceries remained on stripped shelves. Jamie purchased canned goods and breads in preparation for the possibility of a lengthy power outage. Winds picked up. Sheets of driving rain pummeled the windows of their room. Big waves battered the dock. They played in the splash of the crashing surf and took pictures, before hunkering down. Fortunately, neither St. Kitts nor the university suffered any serious damage.

Classes commenced on schedule. Heather and classmate, Lauren, became best friends. Air conditioning didn't exist many places. Year round, perpetual perspiration dampened their nursing student uniforms, sticking the cloth to their skin.

At the city hospital, they assisted women giving birth in a hot room with nothing but a small, portable fan to cool them. Nurse-midwives rendered all prenatal and obstetrical care, including delivering the baby. A doctor participated only when there was a serious complication.

Each patient had a paper chart created, that was tied together with string. Narcotics were rarely administered. Lacking electrical IV pumps, nurses adjusted intravenous drips by counting the number of drops in a minute. Wound care was basic.

Heather and Lauren were the only students who enrolled in the public health course. At community health fairs, they performed sugar and blood-pressure checks for hundreds of Kittitians. Held outdoors in extreme heat, sweat bubbled, forming tiny rivulets that streamed down their skin.

The dedicated young women provided care to psychiatric patients and amputees at the government-funded Cardin Home. Very bleak and without air-conditioning, sparse furnishings added to the building's desolation. It lacked any actual windows and doors.

Instead, unscreened, rectangular openings in its walls of cinder blocks, served the function.

Always hungry for a tasty lunch, Heather said they'd scoot around the corner to the rustic Marlins' Café, very cheap and delicious. The cook specialized in chicken roti or hot dogs topped with mayo, ketchup, and lettuce. Served with hot fries, often he gave the girls a second hot dog in the one bun.

Lauren picks up the St. Kitts story:

"When I first met Heather, I stared at her neck. The puckered tracheotomy scar isn't easily hidden. Her breathy voice waved like a flag begging for inquiries, but maybe answering questions would make her relive a painful experience. People must pester her all the time. Eventually, my curiosity was appeased.

"A nursing instructor asked Heather to tell her story of boundless resilience. Afterward, she showed me the *Woman's Day* article. It seemed impossible! How could Heather be that abandoned baby?

"Heather is one of the most genuine and selfless people whom I have ever known. She envisions a silver lining to any trouble. Despite any frustrations tossed her way, she discovers something to laugh about. She always created fun, even while we struggled with long hours of daunting studies in our apartment.

"Celebrating Heather's twenty-fourth birthday was an amazing day. We boarded the thirty-minute boat ferry to the island of Nevis. We sat on the open deck and gazed out over the clear turquoise water.

"'I hope I see the dolphins this year,' Heather said. I looked puzzled, so she explained. 'On my birthday, they come to see me.' I thought it highly improbable. Numerous times I'd rode the ferry and never seen any.

"Arriving at Nevis, we walked to the beach and swam in the surf. At the Four Seasons hotel, we lounged poolside, ordered a couple of fruity drinks, and jumped into the ice-cold pond at their spa (perfect for the sweltering day).

"Returning on the ferry to St. Kitts, lo and behold, everyone on-board began excitedly yelling in a happy way. I ran out of the snack bar to find out why. Heather motioned me to look over the railing. She pointed to the water churning alongside the boat. Dolphins pumped their powerful tails, speeding along, breaking through the froth to peer up at Heather. Indeed, they had come to see her!"

At the school year's end, I flew there for the formal pinning ceremony. Heather and Lauren spoiled me with a drive through old sugar-cane lands to supper at Sprat Nets, a thatched-roof restaurant next to open fishing waters. As the sun set, we dined on Johnny cakes, grilled fresh-caught lobster, and roasted hot corn on the cob.

Both were accepted to Colorado State University Pueblo for their last year. Academic schedule gave them only one week to move to Colorado Springs. Stuffing what they could into the two-suitcase limit for their flights back to the United States, they had to throw away most of their belongings. To depart St. Kitts, Heather and I chose an overnight layover in Puerto Rico. We strolled along the cobbled streets of old San Juan and meandered past its historic buildings and fortresses.

Heather's few days in Florida were busy, catching up with friends and family. She and Jim talked nonstop about all of her adventures. "I had a patient with a tracheotomy. It was super scary," she told him.

"Funny to experience it from the other side," he commented.

While Heather was away in the islands, Tony married Ashley in a beautiful riverside ceremony. On St. Patrick's Day, the young couple was blessed with a baby girl, Cora Lee. Heather scooped up her niece. We all delighted in Cora. Becoming Grandpa brought great joy to Jim, and his eyes regained a sparkle.

In preparation for the trip to Colorado, Jim showed Heather how to check the oil, brake, and radiator fluids in the ten-year-old Subaru that we'd bought for her. Equipped with all-wheel drive, we hoped it would keep her safe in snowy weather. Heather and I drove the scenic route across the country, stopping to see relatives in Kansas, the buffalo in the Black Hills, and traversed the high roads of Rocky Mountain National Park. My cousin, Sara, and her husband, Rich, took us to bet on the horses at Arapahoe Park outside of Denver. Arriving in Colorado Springs, we lugged all of her belongings to the upstairs apartment that she and Lauren would share.

Their final year of course work and clinical rotations sped by. Heather Giganti and Lauren Delizia graduated from the Colorado State University-Pueblo's College of Nursing in early August of 2012. Jamie and I beamed with pride as the professor handed Heather her diploma at the graduation ceremony. Our hearts soared, riding the glory throughout the weekend of celebration. Heather shed some bittersweet tears as Jim was too ill to attend. He sent his congratulations and wishes for many blessings in the girls' near and distant future.

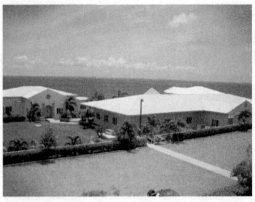

International University of Nursing
St. Kitts

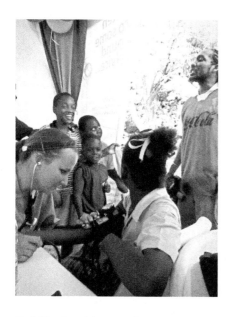
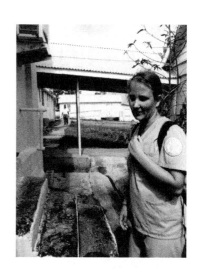

Public Health Nursing

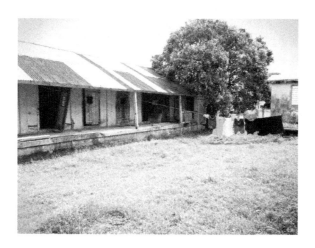

Cardin Home

Ann Widick Giganti

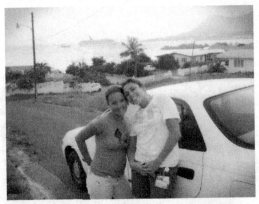

Heather and Lauren leaving St. Kitts for Colorado

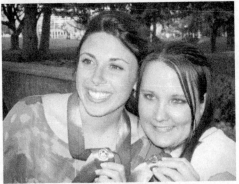

Lauren Delizia and Heather graduating Colorado State University, Pueblo's College of Nursing

Heather left Colorado and drove through Texas to Florida. Young and forever love waited. Matt Lucher declared his love with beach sand.

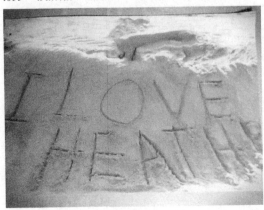

In Florida, on August 28, Matt and Heather strolled to Riverside Park, about a block from our home. Clouds spilled rain. The happy couple splashed through accumulating puddles. Gazing over the lagoon to watch the vibrant sunset, Matt dropped to one knee and proposed marriage. Heather embraced him, answering an ecstatic "Yes." Matt slipped the engagement ring and its exquisite diamonds onto her finger.

CHAPTER 33] NO GUARANTEE

All along, Jim insisted that the children and I enjoy the best of life, even though his poor health hindered him. "No sense you suffering the loss of exuberant adventures, too," he said. Wise and generous, as thus far he'd been sick a dozen years.

Heather deferred applying for her first nursing job until after she and I travelled to India. Family and co-workers would look after Jim. Heather and I could communicate daily by phone, text, or e-mail. We daydreamed that Jim might meet us in Paris, but knew it was an impossible fantasy.

Gujarat, India was the primary destination. I wanted to experience the land and culture of where Mahesh and Rita Soni had grown up, as had many of the other local physicians. An overnight Lufthansa flight landed us in Frankfurt, Germany. Another flight landed us in Delhi. A crowded, wild bus ride took us to northern India.

Heather and I spent three days listening to the Dalai Lama's teachings in his home temple in Dharamshala. Next we went to Delhi to join a temporary tent-city gathering of 1.2 million people of the Nirankari mission, devoted to "Universal Brotherhood, One world, One vast family." Onward, we went to tour Ghandi's ashram in Ahmedabad, home base for the ideology that set India free from Britain.

Next was Sasan Gir National Park, last natural habitat for the Asiatic lions. Only five-hundred remain alive in the world. I snapped photos of lotus flowers, standing on the banks of the Hiran River. A local gained Heather's attention. "Tell your mother that crocodiles are lurking there," he warned.

The cell phone only had service bars outside our windowless hut. Due to the time difference, I called Jim as the sun set. "Dad is going to hear Mom get pounced on by a lion," Heather said.

"I'll prove that I am thriving," Jim said. "Hold on, I'll go step on the scale. Yep, I weigh the same, 155 pounds. I'm fine," Jim insisted.

"Heather and I are going on a jeep safari in the morning, to see the Asiatic lions," I said.

That night, Zulu tribesman, descendants of slaves who had hidden in the forest when the British departed, demonstrated their traditional dances. In the outdoor gathering area, we formed a circle around the performers. Most guests had never seen white people before and warned their children not to talk to the strangers.

A tribesman invited Heather to join in one of the dances. The fearful people laughed at her awkwardness in following the rhythm, high leaps, and deep squats. "Mom, I heard something rip, and I don't think it was my pants." After that, the other guests became friendly to us.

In the morning, the same tribesman, who had danced, tracked the lions to insure that Heather and I would see several from our open jeep tour. The chief protector of the lions was Ajay Ratnaker. "If it comes to choosing between protecting you or the lions; I will protect my lions," he said.

A day's drive, and we were granted permission to tour the medical school that Mahesh Soni attended in Vadodora. I was

315

surprised when my phone rang. It was Dr. Bansal, Jim's pulmonologist. "Your husband is not being truthful. He is dying," he said.

Neither Jim, nor Heather, nor I would get to visit Paris and the Eiffel Tower.

Jim admitted he'd been fibbing; he wanted us to finish our trip. He checked into the local hospital, hoping to survive until we made it back. In preparation to get him home, a friend arranged delivery of an oxygen concentrator, identical to the one that Heather had once used.

On Thanksgiving Day, Heather and I landed in Orlando and checked Jim out of the hospital and got him home to his own bed. The next evening, we all gathered around Tony and Ashley's dining table to eat leftovers. Grandma came too.

A fire blazed in the outdoor pit. Heather and Matt fished off the dock. Jamie and Marcus were home in Seattle. In the past, each time Jamie flew home, at our urging, Jim had always rallied. Cora snuggled up with Jim, and together they watched Disney movies. About midnight, we drove Grandma home.

At sunrise, I awakened and gazed at Jim. He opened his eyes.

"I am not doing well. I can't move, I am gone," he said. For a couple of minutes, his breath entered and exited his body peacefully, then grew heavy. Gathering my wits, I raced down the hallway and woke Heather and Matt.

Heather snuggled her head gently on her dad's dying chest, enfolding her arms around his sickly body. "What do we do?" she asked, tears streaming, looking at him the way he'd beheld her that first time he'd cradled her.

"Nothing. He said he's gone. We let him go. He's suffered long enough," I said. His breath stopped. I let the oxygen concentrator keep running, infusing enriched air to the nasal prongs in Jim's lifeless nose, maintaining an illusion of him sleeping. Turning it off would have created a suffocating quiet.

The saddest call I've ever made was to his mother. I'd known him thirty-seven years, but she'd known him for sixty. Our children had never known life without him.

Grieving, Heather cancelled all wedding plans, postponing the ceremony indefinitely. "Not without my Dad, I don't want to get married without my father," Heather insisted. The statement was compatible with her emotions, yet crazy as her requirement could never be met.

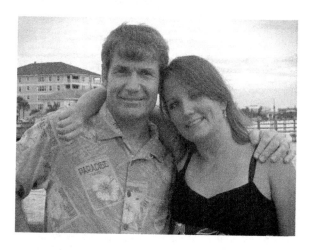

Heather and the best father ever, Jim Giganti

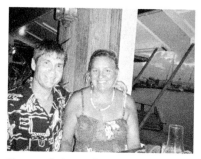

Jim and Ann Giganti

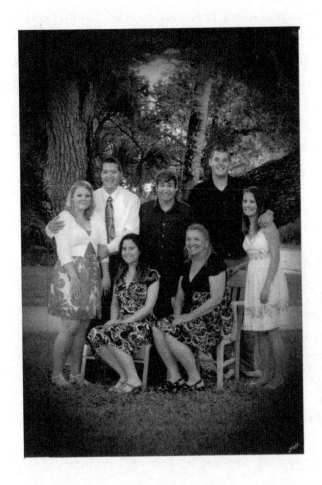

Giganti family 2011 (all except Marcus). Front: Jamie and Ann.
Back: Ashley, Tony, Jim, Matt, Heather

SURPRISE

Heather was offered an RN job as a night nurse on the cancer floor at North Florida Regional Medical Center in Gainesville. She and Matt rented a nearby apartment. Late in June, Heather drove to Indialantic to help me empty everything out of the home that Jim and I had shared for so many years. After his death, I'd discovered that I didn't want to live there without him.

Something had been paining Heather's abdomen. She thought she had an obstruction as a consequence of the many surgeries she'd undergone as a baby. I ordered an ultrasound of her belly.

"It is not a tumor. Are you happy?" the technician asked us.

Long scars had compressed her growing uterus and prevented any telltale bulge. Surprise! She was six and one-half month's pregnant, and the infant was positioned breech. Heather and Matt were expecting a daughter. The forthcoming calls that she made were exhilarating and comical.

Truth be told, Heather thought she was badly constipated. Matt said he was going to tell their child that her momma thought she was poop.

One week later, Matt accompanied her to the first appointment with the obstetrician. Another surprise, this one more terrifying, an ambulance transferred Heather to Shands. She was admitted to the high-risk labor and delivery unit. The bag of amniotic fluid had almost slipped out of her body. Enclosed within the bulging membranes, the baby's foot was also dangerously dangling down.

Two weeks later, Lilly was delivered by emergency caesarian section. Born twelve weeks early, she weighed two pounds and thirteen ounces. Walking the steps to the neonatal intensive care unit to see her, I about had a panic attack. Please, not again. I did not want to traverse the path that we had with Heather, nor one that was more dismal.

Lilly's troubles were not as severe as what Heather had experienced, but she had close-call scares. Heather and Matt carried most of the burden. Once she could be out of the incubator, tiny, wrinkled baby Lilly looked as small as a peanut cradled on Matt's chest. As tough a fighter as her mom, at five pounds, Lilly went home.

A job opened up at Shands Hospital in the pediatric intensive care unit. Employment scheduled an interview for Heather to meet the nurse supervisor. "Didn't you reside here as a baby? I used to care for you," she stated.

Heather finds it tremendously rewarding to work in the same PICU where she first lived.

Eighteen months later, I'd saved up some money. "Heather, does Matt still want to marry you?" I questioned.

"I think so, I'll go ask him." Matt confirmed that he did. They set the date for August 8th. We set to planning the wedding.

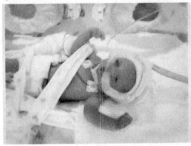

Lillian James Lucher, July 22, 2013

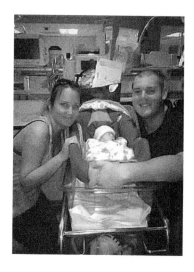

Heather, Lilly, Matt

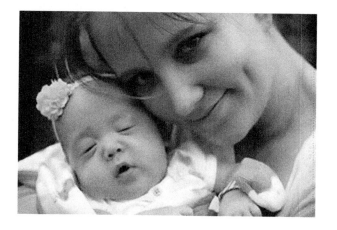

Lilly and Heather

CHAPTER 34] HAPPY ENDING

The wedding. That Saturday, rain poured all day until an hour before the ceremony. Many friends prayed the torrents would stop. The downpour kept everything cool for an August 8 hot Florida summer day. Guests took their seats under a thatched-roof gazebo overlooking the ocean.

Joy filled my heart. The delight is indescribable as I looked at radiant Heather on the arm of her brother, Tony. She stumbled walking on the wooden planks, and he caught her. Both giggled. Tall, handsome Matt waited. Their miracle daughter, Lilly, adorned with lavender ribbons in her hair, stood quietly next to beautiful Jamie. Jim's mom sat in the first folding chair.

The minister bestowed their vows. Matt carried his bride inside to the ballroom for a catered reception, DJ, and dancing. Tony's wife, Ashley, had arranged beautiful decorations of shells, starfish, and roses. Dawn, photographer and friend, had the newlyweds pose on the sandy beach for photos with their daughter. Our good friend, Sudarshan, sang a blessing in Hindi. Then we all danced, and danced some more. Joy and happiness effervesced throughout the evening's celebration of love.

Heather, I thank you for a journey impossible to envision that day you summoned me. How clearly I remember silent crying and that when our eyes met, your soul captured mine. Dad melted the moment he cradled you as a sickly baby against his chest. Instantly and forever you charmed Jamie's heart, starting with your impish study of the black-winged bug that lighted upon your wrist. Tony loved you long before he raced out the front door with a wagon full of toys that first time he welcomed you home.

Thanks, Heather, for picking us to be your family, and to all who touched our lives and made possible the miracle of Heather. A special recognition goes out to Dr. Bruce Maddern, the surgeon whose hands gave Heather the gifts of voice and the joy of swimming with the dolphins.

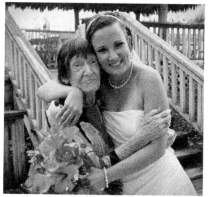

Heather and her Grandma Jean

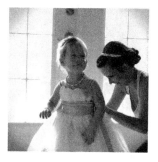

Heather and daughter, Lilly

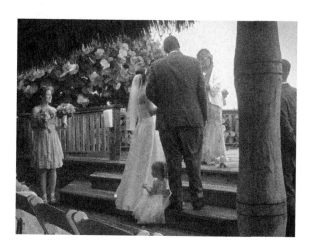

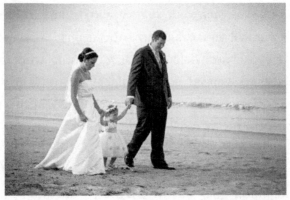

Mr. and Mrs. Lucher and daughter Lilly

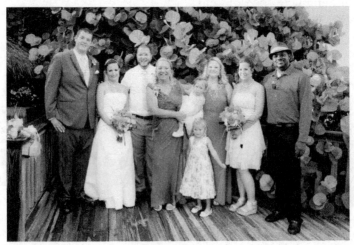

Giganti Family
Matt, Heather, Tony, Ann, Lilly, Cora, Ashley, Jamie, Marcus

"Giving thanks every day. Giving thanks every way."
--the end--

Printed in Great Britain
by Amazon

39304923R00185